The Growing Global Public Health Crisis
and how to address it

DAVID H STONE

Professor of Paediatric Epidemiology, University of Glasgow, UK

Foreword by
Sir Michael Marmot, Director,
UCL Institute of Health Equity

Radcliffe Publishing
London • New York

Radcliffe Publishing Ltd
33–41 Dallington Street
London
EC1V 0BB
United Kingdom

www.radcliffepublishing.com

British Library Cataloguing in Publication Data

A catalogue record for this book is available from the British Library.

ISBN-13: 978 1 84619 471 9

Typeset by Phoenix Photosetting, Chatham, Kent, UK
Cover designed by Cox Design Ltd, Witney, Oxon, UK
Printed and bound by Cadmus Communications, USA

Contents

Foreword

In 1978 the public health world was inspired by the Alma Ata declaration of Health for All, through primary healthcare. But the inspiration only went so far. A senior Canadian colleague said that, at the time, a common reaction in high-income countries was: Primary care? We are developing tertiary care; there's nothing in this for us.

Regrettably, there is still a great deal of such thinking. Global public health is seen by many as focused on the problems of low-income countries. Rich countries have different problems: mental illness, non-communicable disease, ageing and associated frailties and disability. In this way of thinking, there is therefore little overlap between the necessary approaches to public health in high- and low-income countries. I have left middle-income countries out of this caricature because, as anyone who has looked at the evidence knows, overwhelmingly their health problems are coming to resemble those of high-income countries.

There is no doubt that there are considerable health problems associated with poverty in low-income countries. David Stone cites some statistics:

➤ 10 000 babies die every day in the world before they are four weeks old
➤ over 500 000 women die in childbirth each year
➤ more than 750 000 children die every year of measles
➤ 1.6 million people die in the world every year of tuberculosis.

It is a fair judgement that this appalling toll of mortality should be largely preventable. The limitation is not lack of biological understanding of why these deaths occur. The problems are social, political, economic and cultural, not ignorance of biomedical science. This is where public health should come in. What is needed is knowledge of a different sort – how to organise to take action to solve these problems. Given that these preventable problems persist, this other kind of knowledge – organising to take action – is key.

The present book presents a thorough and systematic account of public health in a global arena. At first blush, it might seem that there is no continuity between the approach needed to address this unnecessary toll of diseases of poverty and that needed for the problems of non-communicable disease in middle- and high-income countries. The strength of David Stone's book is that he lays out a set of principles and approaches that should have general applicability to all public health problems wherever we find them. Personally, I have been fighting the fight on social determinants of health. Improving public health is not 'simply' a matter of technical solutions. Technical solutions are vital, of course. They address causes of disease. The mantra underlying the social determinants of health is to address the causes of the causes.

The need is great. To the social problems of preventable ill health we must add the challenges of climate change and environmental damage; the political problems of violence and civil unrest; the social problems of discrimination and exclusion.

David Stone's guidelines start from a similar viewpoint but his book then goes into the principles not only of what to do but how to go about it. But, argues Stone, before we approach the public health equivalents of diagnosis and cure, we need shared values and an overarching vision on where we are going and what we would like to achieve. I agree, as I agree with his call for use of evidence to underpin our strategies.

I particularly like Stone's challenges for the future:
➤ investigate and promote wellbeing, mental health and quality of life
➤ nurture salutogenesis, including boosting social capital, resilience and resistance
➤ seek professional mechanisms to balance human rights and responsibilities
➤ confront violence, terrorism and conflict as public health challenges
➤ exploit more fully the public health role of healthcare systems and practitioners
➤ resolve the tension between competing public health objectives.

The combination of theoretical understanding, recognition of the importance of values, reliance on evidence and practical guides for action makes this book a welcome contribution to the practice of global public health.

Sir Michael Marmot
UCL Institute of Health Equity
December 2011

Preface

First, two disclaimers: this is neither a reference text on global health, of which there are several fine examples in existence, nor is it an academic review of its achievements and deficiencies. Indeed, it is not an academic text, in the conventional sense, at all but is rather a kind of extended essay. It expresses a highly personal, perhaps idiosyncratic view about the nature of the global public health narrative of the early 21st century, the manner in which intellectual debates tend to be being framed around it, and potentially fruitful avenues for exploring fresh strategic thinking about global public health.

The book is aimed at a global multidisciplinary readership in public health, both academic and professional, working in fields as diverse as epidemiology, environmental health, communicable disease control, health promotion, healthcare management, injury and violence prevention, international health and policy development. It will, in addition, help to serve the educational needs of both undergraduates and postgraduates in the wider healthcare and related fields. It will also appeal to a broad, general (non-professional or academic) readership that is curious about the world and its current state of health.

As I describe more fully in the Introduction, public health professionals assess population health in an analogous way to their clinical colleagues. They assess the presenting symptoms and signs, undertake a few further tests and reach a diagnosis (even if it is a tentative one) by integrating all of this information. That is what Section 1 of the book is about. By the time you have finished reading it, you will have a fairly clear idea of the global public health 'diagnosis', or the state of health of the world's population, and whether or not you endorse my use of the 'crisis' epithet. Section 2 will take that diagnosis as its starting point and set about identifying 'treatment' strategies, comprising principles and action points, for addressing it. Section 3 outlines the necessary 'follow-up' measures to ensure that the interventions are working effectively, efficiently and transparently, and to scan the horizon for newly emerging challenges.

The word 'crisis' is undeniably overused. In common parlance, it means a critical juncture or turning point and implies that decisive action is necessary to resolve it and thereby avert a serious threat. The term has also been invoked in a medical context to denote either a sudden change in the course of a disease or fever, toward either improvement or deterioration, or an emotionally stressful event or traumatic change in a person's life. All of these meanings are relevant to the content of this book.

Readers will note that, although I have appended the core elements of a possible 'horizontal' global public health strategy, I offer no grandiose guaranteed blueprints for solving the world's public health problems. That would be as rash as a clinician claiming an ability to solve an individual's health problems by prescribing a guaranteed cure. Nevertheless, like clinical medicine, public health now has at its disposal a formidable armamentarium of evidence-based responses that, if applied appropriately, can make significant inroads into population health. Despite its title, this book is firmly, if cautiously, optimistic. Human ingenuity has repeatedly risen to the challenges of history. With a combination of intellectual rigour, clarity of vision, political will and a modicum of good luck, there is no reason why it should not do so again in response to the global public health crisis.

About the author

David H Stone is a public health physician and researcher based in Glasgow University's Paediatric Epidemiology and Community Health (PEACH) Unit, which he founded in 1995. He has had a long-standing commitment to child health in general and injury prevention in particular. He has held academic appointments at St Thomas' Hospital, London, Ben Gurion University of the Negev, Israel, and Glasgow University, where he has held a Personal Chair of Paediatric Epidemiology since 2000. He chaired the Child Injury Group of the Accidental Injury Task Force of the UK Department of Health and was Chair of the International Society for Child and Adolescent Injury Prevention, 2000–2003.

Acknowledgements

Many people gave me the encouragement and practical help that proved so necessary to propel this book from conception to completion. In particular, I am grateful to my endlessly patient secretary, Rita Dobbs, who protected me from the intrusions of the real world of work during my writing time; to my PEACH Unit colleagues, Krista Kleinberg and Mhairi Campbell, whose eagle eyes greatly enhanced the quality of the text; and to the countless students and colleagues of all nationalities who have, over many years, convinced me that global public health is of paramount importance to us all.

Abbreviations

ACE	Adverse childhood experience
AIDS	Acquired immune deficiency syndrome
APHA	American Public Health Association
BMI	Body Mass Index
CBA	Cost–benefit analysis
CEA	Cost–effectiveness analysis
CUA	Cost–utility analysis
DALY	Disability-adjusted life-year
DFLE	Disability-free life expectancy
DSM-IV	*Diagnostic and Statistical Manual of Mental Disorders*, 4th edition
DT	Demographic transition
EBM	Evidence-based medicine
ED	Emergency department
ET	Epidemiological transition
FPH	Faculty of Public Health
GBD	Global burden of disease
GEC	Global environmental change
GNP	Gross national product
HALE	Health-Adjusted Life Expectancy
HIV	Human immunodeficiency virus
IMF	International Monetary Fund
IPCC	Intergovernmental Panel on Climate Change
MDG	Millennium Development Goal
NCD	Non-communicable disease
NGO	Non-governmental organisation
NHS	National Health Service
NICE	National Institute for Health and Clinical Excellence
QALY	Quality-adjusted life-year
RCT	Randomised controlled trial
RTC	Road traffic crash
RTI	Road traffic injury
SOC	Sense of coherence

ST	Sustainability transition
TB	Tuberculosis
UK	United Kingdom
UN	United Nations
UNICEF	United Nations Children's Fund
US	United States (of America)
WHA	World Health Assembly
WHO	World Health Organization
YLD	Years of life lived (lost) with disability
YLL	Years of life lost

Introduction: the nature of global public health

In coming years, our societies won't face one or two major challenges at once ... they'll face an alarming variety of problems all at the same time. (Thomas Homer-Dixon)

The future of public health is to continue to make a difference in conditions in the broader international community. The challenge is to adapt our public health strategy to control environments and modify behaviours in a constantly changing world. Even with the expertise of modern medicine, people in the industrialised world may be surprised to find that they are woefully unprepared for the far-reaching challenges of an impending large-scale public health catastrophe. (Steven M Wolinsky)

This book is about the current state of global health and the huge challenge that it poses to every nation on earth. It contains both an epidemiological overview of the key problems and an account of some key evidence-based public health solutions, including a proposed global public health strategy with recommended actions ranked, where possible, in order of approximate priority.

Readers will quickly discover that the book has been written from a strategic public health perspective. Its underlying premise is that such a perspective is logical, necessary and highly productive as a means of generating fresh thinking about how we might act to protect and improve the health of the world's population. If that premise is wrong or unclear, the remainder of the book will teeter unsteadily atop the shakiest of foundations. To minimise that risk, I set out in these introductory pages my understanding of what is meant by global public heath and how I have used the concept to construct the book.

Apart from the word 'health', there is unquestionably a strong connection, though not necessarily a seamless one, between the three endeavours described as public health, international health and global health respectively. A fourth term – global public health – is a kind of amalgam of all three. It is worth briefly reviewing what these various terms mean as they are not always used synonymously.

WHAT IS PUBLIC HEALTH?

We may think we know what public health is but it turns out that perhaps we don't – or rather that one person's idea of what constitutes public health may be very different from another's. One source of confusion is that the field has been rapidly changing over the last few decades. In the United Kingdom, for example, where I have spent most of my professional life, the term virtually disappeared with the reorganisation of the National Health Service in 1974. Prior to that date, public health was largely and, by most accounts, unsatisfactorily located in local authorities (a setting to which, ironically, it seems set to return in the 21st century). Its replacement was called 'community medicine' – a term that turned out to be a serious misnomer as the specialty was neither community based nor a purely medical discipline, and was quietly discarded after a few years. We should therefore try to banish any terminological vagueness before proceeding further.

The term 'public health' appears, at first sight, to mean 'the health of the public' or 'population health'. Neither of those phrases fully encapsulates the concept. Some readers may associate public health with engineering programmes to supply clean water and remove sewage from overcrowded towns and cities. That was true, in part at least, of the Victorian era and still has great relevance in the world's poorest regions but it is an inadequate stereotype that barely accords with the reality of public health in the 21st century. Others may believe that public health strives to obliterate epidemics of infectious diseases, or change patterns of unhealthy behaviour, or create safer, healthier environments for children, or organise and administer healthcare systems, or perform research on the frequency, causes and prevention of disease. All these notions tell us something about the public health project but they fail, either separately or collectively, to tell the whole story.

Definitions of health and public health

Public health is far from easy to define in a manner that satisfies everyone. One reason for this is that *health* itself is a subtle, abstract concept. In 1946, the World Health Organization (1974) defined health as: 'a state of complete physical, mental and social wellbeing and not merely the absence of disease or infirmity'.

That statement is so familiar today that we tend to underestimate its ingenuity. Well ahead of its time, it emphasised positive health rather than the presence of disease, and attempted to integrate physical, mental and social dimensions into a single entity. These were both relatively novel ideas. And the inclusion of wellbeing (a component of quality of life) in the definition initially attracted minimal attention but turned out to be farsighted. The concept of wellbeing has, in recent years, been recognised as an important dimension of health that is stimulating intensive research. At the same time, the definition has been subjected to criticism on various grounds: that it represents an unattainable ideal state, that it implies a static rather than a dynamic phenomenon, and that it is individualistic rather than collective (to cite just three). Subsequent attempts to amend it have tended merely to confuse matters. It speaks volumes for the shrewdness of the original authors that it remains the only definition to command a degree of universal acquiescence, if not enthusiasm, after more than six decades.

There is no internationally agreed definition of *public health* but rather several competing versions that co-exist in a kind of permanent truce. Its most basic (and nebulous) meaning is the cluster of cognate fields that are concerned with the prevention of disease and the promotion of health. It is also used to indicate a preoccupation with the health of whole populations and communities rather than individuals. The Faculty of Public Health (FPH), the main standard-setting organisation for the multidisciplinary specialty of public health in the UK, borrowing heavily from the early 20th-century writings of the American bacteriologist and public health pioneer Winslow, and reiterated by the Acheson Committee (Department of Health 1988), defines public health as: 'The science and art of promoting and protecting health and well-being, preventing ill-health and prolonging life through the organised efforts of society' (www.fph.org.uk/what_is_public_health).

Several features of the FPH definition are noteworthy and pertinent to the arguments presented in this book. First, it indicates that public health is not merely a scientific pursuit but one that also involves a set of attributes that lie in the realm of human creativity and judgement; these 'soft' skills may together be described as constituting the 'art' component. Second, prolonging life is neither the sole nor even primary aim of public health; improving quality of life is the unwritten subtext. Third, preventing disease and promoting health are complementary though not identical activities since the latter encompasses efforts to enhance positive health and wellbeing rather than merely to interrupt pathological processes. Fourth, public health is a systematic, societal activity rather than the sum total of a series of one-off initiatives that may be undertaken with similar aims, by individuals or organisations. Finally, the definition is an inclusive one that embraces practice, policy making and research across a wide range of disciplines, most of which do not include the term 'public health' in their titles. Nor does it exclude individualistic healthcare, though an earlier version of the FPH definition implied that it did, by appending a phrase, since dropped, referring to 'populations rather than individuals'. This was an explicit attempt to distance public health from clinical practice.

This last point is much more important – and controversial – than it may appear at first sight. Even today, many public health professionals prefer to view their work as being exclusively population based and resist being drawn into 'clinical' or other activities that are aimed at individuals. In reality, a population is always composed of individuals and the distinction is largely a theoretical or ideological one. Furthermore, much public health involves the delivery of interventions (including immunisation and screening) to large numbers of individuals with the close collaboration of clinicians whose participation is essential to the process. This topic has generated fairly heated debate around the true nature of public health and, in particular, its relationship to clinical practice.

Though this may seem a somewhat pedantic point, public health and health promotion are not synonymous. Health promotion is (arguably) a narrower concept than public health. Despite efforts by the WHO and others to broaden it, health promotion tends to emphasise behavioural change as the key to health improvement. Here is a typical definition of health promotion: 'the science and art of helping people change their lifestyle to move toward a state of optimal health' (Minkler 1989).

A key point to remember is that 'public health', in the sense used here, is synonymous with neither 'the health of the public' nor 'the health of the population'. Rather, public health is the professional and organisational *response* – in terms of resources and action – to deal with the challenges posed by population health. The state of population heath, as assessed epidemiologically, is the problem while 'public health' seeks to offer the solution. When a population or group finds itself in a state of severe distress, as manifested epidemiologically by unacceptably high mortality or morbidity rates, an obligation to offer appropriate and effective countermeasures falls upon the professionals and agencies charged with explicit responsibility to prevent disease and promote health. To put it another way, if there is a global crisis in public health, as this book suggests, the burden of responsibility for its genesis may be traced primarily to our collective failure to act decisively to confront it rather than to any characteristics, actions or obstacles originating within the population itself. To suggest that responsibility for the problem lies with the population – or to the individuals who comprise it – amounts to a kind of aggregate victim blaming that is as unhelpful as it is unfair.

The enlarging scope of public health

Public health, as we know it today, evolved from the social reform movements in 19th-century Europe and North America. The pioneering work of Farr, Chadwick, Snow, Virchow, Koch, Simon and others demonstrated that taking effective action to improve health was not exclusively dependent on a detailed understanding of the biological mechanisms of disease causation. They showed how much could be achieved by observing and documenting the pattern of disease in the population, drawing inferences about its spread, designing practical countermeasures and monitoring the impact of interventions. The embryonic discipline of epidemiology became as important to the detection, management and prevention of outbreaks and epidemics of infectious diseases as the laboratory-based sciences of bacteriology, virology and parasitology. Inevitably, these twin approaches became closely intertwined and achieved considerable success in communicable disease control.

Although public health was originally highly focused on the identification and control of infectious diseases, its remit steadily widened in the 20th century to include the identification and control of risk factors for chronic disease, along with the medical management of health services. This led to the forging of a natural alliance with physicians, administrators and a wide range of other healthcare professionals. More recently, following the publication of landmark documents such as the Lalonde Report (Lalonde 1974), the Alma-Ata Declaration (World Health Organization 1978) and the Ottawa Declaration (World Health Organization 1986), public health has again reoriented itself towards more broadly based, holistic approaches that address upstream influences on health and disease, a trend that has been characterised by some writers as the 'new public health'.

Nowadays, the key goal of public health in most countries is perceived to be health improvement (implemented through the linked but discrete fields of health promotion, health protection and disease prevention) and is undertaken by a multidisciplinary workforce. Yet the discipline is still evolving. A recent UK reformulation of public health action reiterates this view and adds to its remit *the reduction in health inequalities* (Skills for Health 2002), reflecting the growing preoccupation of both the public health community and government of that country with the diverging health fortunes of the rich and the poor. Implicit in this new objective is presumably the aspiration to improve the health of disadvantaged sectors rather than to lower the health of more privileged communities (though the latter would also theoretically reduce health inequality). McMichael and Beaglehole (2009), responding to the green agenda, have called for the inclusion of a further dimension – striving for *life-supporting and health-sustaining natural, social and economic environments*.

These recent elaborations arguably verge on the tautological and contribute little to our understanding of the fundamental goal of public health – to protect and improve the health of the population. They may also unnecessarily complicate the task of explaining to the general public – and to the ranks of public health practitioners and students – what the field is about. Nevertheless, they deserve serious attention as they are becoming such prominent features of the modern public health movement and may turn out to be important motivators of the new generation of its practitioners.

INTERNATIONAL HEALTH, GLOBAL HEALTH AND GLOBAL PUBLIC HEALTH

We have established that public health is an idea, a way of looking at and responding to health problems at a population level. But what exactly is meant by the term 'global public health' and how does it relate to 'international health' and 'global health'? They are often used interchangeably but some writers have suggested that there are distinctions to be drawn between them. All of them share some key characteristics: they seek to base decisions on epidemiological data and evidence, they focus on populations, groups and communities, they value social justice and equity, and they emphasise prevention.

International health has been defined in various ways, ranging from the practice of medicine in developing countries to all forms of public health and healthcare that cross national boundaries. One of the clearest definitions is that of Sharma and Atri (2010): 'The science and art of examining health problems in multiple countries, primarily those that are developing, and finding population-based solutions to their problems'.

Global health goes a step further conceptually than international health. It views the earth and its health as a single interconnected whole rather than merely the sum of its individual regions and countries. This is a paradigm shift that implies the need for a collective, transnational analysis and response to international health challenges. The notion of a global dimension to human affairs (including health) is not new but was once considered either a theoretical abstraction or a kind of idealised and probably unachievable aspiration, mainly because of the complexity, diversity and sheer scale of thinking required to view the world, in all its variety and complexity, as a single entity.

There are obvious dangers in seeking to generalise in any meaningful way about the entire population of the world. The health problems of Botswana are very different from those of Brazil. That objection expresses a variant of the epidemiological fallacy – observations in the population as a whole do not necessarily apply to individuals. The existence of the epidemiological fallacy does not negate the value of epidemiology as a scientific method. Similarly, adopting a global perspective on population health enables us to discern patterns that would otherwise be invisible if we confined the observations to single countries or communities. But there is a risk that we draw conclusions and prescribe solutions that will not always suit every country. So we should be aware of the dangers of generalisation without being paralysed into inertia by that awareness.

As with all forms of epidemiology, time trends can intrude to complicate the picture. None of the relevant parameters of global health has remained static in the last half century. On the contrary, the world's population has increased, its industrial and agricultural activity has been radically transformed, and its geopolitical landscape has changed beyond recognition. Yet, paradoxically, the use of the 'global' epithet has become more relevant than ever, its ubiquity reinforced in our generation by the rapid advances in communications technology, particularly the internet, which have enormously enhanced our capacity for international information exchange, collaborative research, training and practice, and political co-ordination.

Koplan *et al* (2009) emphasise the collaborative and collective nature of global health in their conceptualisation of the discipline as an area for study, research and practice that places a priority on improving health and achieving equity in health for all people worldwide. They view global health as a field that highlights transnational health issues, determinants and solutions, involves many disciplines within and beyond the health sciences, promotes interdisciplinary collaboration, and integrates population-based prevention with individual-level clinical care

In drawing a distinction between international health and global health, they argue that global health need not always have an explicitly international dimension. They propose that global health should not refer solely to health-related issues that literally cross international borders. In their view, 'global' refers to the scope of problems, not their location, and denotes any health issue that concerns more than one country or is influenced by transnational factors, such as climate change or urbanisation, or interventions such as polio eradication. Like public health – but unlike international health – global health can focus on domestic health patterns as well as cross-border threats. While epidemic infectious diseases such as dengue, influenza A (H5NI) and HIV infection are clearly global, global health should also address tobacco control, micronutrient deficiencies, obesity, injury prevention, migrant worker health and migration of healthcare practititioners.

For the purposes of this book, *global public health* is regarded as the collective application of the public health approach to the health challenges that confront the world as a whole. Implicit within that definition is a recognition that a collaborative effort is required, in a manner that transcends national and regional boundaries, to analyse and respond to the public health problems confronting all the people of the world.

WHAT IS THE PUBLIC HEALTH APPROACH?

It is often said that an effective corporate or national response to a disease demands a public health approach. What does this mean? At one level, it simply proposes the adoption of a whole-population perspective that depends on epidemiology as its underpinning science, though not at the expense of other potentially helpful disciplinary methods such as genetics, physiology, pharmacology, biochemistry, sociology, statistics, psychology, engineering and ergonomics. But the public health approach also implies a more proactive approach involving the application of a sophisticated and systematic analysis of highly complex health problems, followed by an evidence-based response. The public health approach may be described as the combination of an inquiring yet critical mindset, allied with a set of (mainly epidemiological) scientific techniques, designed to identify and solve health problems occurring in the population.

The public health system, where it exists, is there to fulfil the three basic roles, broadly labelled health promotion, health protection and disease prevention, outlined earlier. As far as the general public is concerned, the second of these is probably paramount. The bare minimum a community or country expects from its public health infrastructure is to be able to identify and ward off any serious threats to the lives and wellbeing of its citizens. Those threats may take a variety of forms but are conventionally perceived to comprise, in the main, infectious disease outbreaks or epidemics, or acute episodes of environmental (mainly air, water, soil or food) pollution. This is an excessively narrow view of health protection. In fact, taking a cue from the WHO definition, any physical, psychological or social factor that causes disease or disability, or that undermines (or threatens to undermine) the wellbeing of a population, should be viewed as a health threat to which a vigorous public health response is merited.

Although the function of public health is, primarily, to identify and counter any form of threat to the health of the population, the degree to which it fulfils this remit is extremely variable within and between countries. The idea of a simple stimulus–response relationship between the appearance of a health threat and the mounting of an intervention to counter it may be appealing but rarely reflects reality. That is because either the stimulus may not initially be recognised or understood, or the response may be unavailable, inadequate or ineffective. We dare not leave this process to the vagaries of chance. Instead, we need to conceptualise and mobilise a more reliable and sophisticated sequence of public health assessment, action and evaluation.

First, we need to recognise that the threat exists. That cannot be taken for granted in the absence of surveillance or other ways of bringing it to professional and public attention. Second, we need to understand the nature, scale, cause and impact of the threat before we can launch a practical and appropriate countermeasure. Third, we need some means of knowing whether the intervention has worked. These three steps, analogous to the clinical tasks of diagnosis, treatment and follow-up, comprise the essential public health response to any disease or other threat to health in the population. To understand the nature of these three steps, we need to explore their components in more detail.

The public health approach: six questions

The public health approach has evolved rapidly over the past century and a half, a relatively short period in the span of human history. It involves adopting a considered, systematic mode of thinking that is both population based and seeks to find solutions to health challenges. Public health is a highly complex and sophisticated multidisciplinary enterprise that involves the performance of a series of sequential tasks that attempt to answer six questions.

1　What is the problem (nature, scale, consequences and costs)?
2　What are its key determinants (risk factors and causes)?
3　What interventions are known to be effective in addressing it (evidence-based prevention or management)?
4　What interventions are actually being applied to address it (implementation)?
5　How effectively and efficiently are these interventions being implemented (audit of measures of known efficacy, or evaluation of measures of unknown efficacy)?
6　What needs to be done to improve and monitor current implementation (recommendations for action)?

These six questions may be rearticulated and subsumed under three headings or steps: needs assessment ('diagnosis'), population-wide intervention ('treatment') and evaluation or monitoring ('follow-up'). The three steps represent the basic tasks of public health professionals and are analogous to the clinical approach to health problems that individual patients present to doctors and other healthcare practitioners.

1　*Needs assessment* ('diagnosis'): what are the nature, scale and determinants of the problem in the population?
2　*Population-wide intervention* ('treatment'): what can be and is being done to address the problem?
3　*Evaluation or monitoring* ('follow-up'): how well are interventions currently being implemented and how might they be improved?

Step 1: needs assessment ('diagnosis')

This involves the analysis and interpretation of epidemiological data, whether these are obtained from routine statistical sources, disease surveillance systems or *ad hoc* surveys. It provides the public health practitioner with an indication of need or a *community diagnosis*. Getting this right is crucial as everything else will flow from it. A greater degree of epidemiological sophistication is required at this stage than is commonly recognised.

The key elements of the process that will inform the community diagnosis are:

➤ clear specification and quantification of the problem or disorder under scrutiny (numerator)
➤ accurate delineation of an appropriate population under study (denominator)
➤ competent application of statistically and epidemiologically robust techniques for calculating and presenting rates or other data (analysis)

➤ drawing valid conclusions about the problem and its impact over time (analogous to unravelling the 'natural history' of a disease) and how it might be addressed (interpretation).

None of the above is straightforward. Apart from the formidable technical challenges of identifying appropriate numerators and denominators, the epidemiologist must decide on the level of detail (in terms of age, gender, socio-economic position, place of residence, diagnosis and a range of other variables) necessary to characterise the population. Once the numbers, ratios, rates or other indicators have been calculated, their interpretation requires the application of specialised statistical and analytical techniques. And as in clinical medicine, the epidemiological diagnosis may sometimes be obscure, imprecise and multifaceted. It may be provisional initially and only become clearer as new data emerge. Interested readers can discover the details of how to conduct such investigations in standard epidemiological texts.

Step 2: population-wide intervention ('treatment')

The second step in the public health approach involves a distillation of the research evidence to *identify efficacious interventions*, combined with a review of what is actually being done in practice. This evidence about efficacy (what has been shown to work using rigorous research methods) is generated by academic departments, research institutes and specialist centres. They do this by undertaking detailed and carefully planned investigations, often in the form of experiments of various types, including randomised controlled trials. Because the quality of published research studies is so variable, a particular type of research evaluation known as *critical appraisal* has been developed for this purpose. Critical appraisal of the scientific literature is the linchpin of evidence-based practice. Its techniques are helpful both in assessing individual reports or papers and in summarising the current state of research evidence pertaining to a particular intervention through systematic reviews and meta-analyses.

Once the evidence base has been scrutinised in this way and practical measures selected for implementation, the next task is to plan and create appropriately funded and supported mechanisms for the effective delivery of those measures to the target population. This critical stage is often neglected in public health with the result that good intentions are never realised because recommendations for action, however meticulously crafted, are not properly implemented.

The public health literature conceptualises intervention to improve, promote and protect health in various ways. One of the most popular is the traditional *three levels of prevention*. This approach has its critics but usefully encapsulates the wide range of preventive measures that may be applied at different points in the natural history (course) of the targeted condition. Prevention may be primary, secondary or tertiary.

Primary prevention

Primary prevention is directed at the *pre-pathogenesis* phase of a disease – that is, before tissue damage has occurred. It is often synonymous with health improvement, promotion and protection. It involves the removal of circumstances, risks and hazards that lead to disease or injury, or the nurturing of individuals, families and communities in ways that protect and improve health. Primary prevention overlaps with the concept of *salutogenesis*, a term coined by Antonovsky (1979) to describe the process of generating health, the mirror image of pathogenesis (the process of generating disease).

Primary prevention includes:

➤ anti-poverty, social inclusion and other polices designed to address material, social and emotional deprivation policies including the creation of appropriate, affordable and salutogenic residential, educational and recreational environments
➤ creation of safe, crime-free and mutually supportive communities, localities and regions through the use of community-based partnerships between statutory and other agencies, legislation (and its enforcement) and other means
➤ physical, mental and social health improvement and protection policies such as immunisation programmes, efforts to optimise diet and nutrition, and action to minimise alcohol consumption and drug misuse, particularly in children and young adults
➤ leisure, sport and other exercise-promoting policies that often have an anti-obesity objective as well as general benefits for health and wellbeing
➤ economic and fiscal measures designed to improve prosperity, achievement, self-esteem, health and wellbeing, including a reduction in health inequalities
➤ sustainable transport, economic, employment, tourism and other policies designed to reduce environmental pollution and address climate change.

Secondary prevention

Secondary prevention focuses on minimising the extent of tissue damage by intervening early in *pathogenesis*. It involves the reduction of disease severity in an established pathogenic process. Secondary prevention often involves early diagnosis and/or treatment (or prevention) of a disorder (or risk of a disorder) that has already become established. The most widely used type of secondary prevention is screening, or the early detection of disease or risk through the examination of populations or groups.

Secondary prevention includes:

➤ screening for diseases (such as congenital anomalies, growth retardation, high blood pressure and postnatal depression) that can lead to earlier diagnosis and treatment, with consequent improved prognosis

➤ screening for risk factors for disease (such as high cholesterol, dietary deficiency and infectious agents) with a view to earlier intervention and a reduced probability of established disease

➤ the wearing of car seatbelts, bicycle helmets and other safety devices to minimise trauma to human tissue in the event of a crash.

Tertiary prevention

Tertiary prevention seeks to alter the *post-pathogenesis* or recovery phase by mitigating the impact of tissue damage rather than preventing it. It involves providing the optimal treatment and rehabilitation to affected individuals to minimise the consequences of the disease, though it prevents neither the occurrence nor the progression of the disease.

Tertiary prevention includes:

➤ administration of effective first aid when an illness or injury first occurs

➤ rapid and skilled emergency service deployment followed by evacuation of ill or injured patients to specialist care facilities

➤ prompt surgery, intensive care and follow-up in hospital and at home

➤ provision of remedial and support services for disabled people.

Step 3: evaluation or monitoring ('follow-up')

The third and final public health step demands an evaluation, audit or monitoring mechanism to determine the effectiveness along with the strengths and weaknesses of current interventions with a view to making recommendations for the future. This is probably the least well understood and hence most neglected aspect of public health. What follows is a bird's eye view of a vast subject.

Evaluation, audit and monitoring are conceptually related terms. Evaluation simply means 'to determine the value of' though it is commonly used to describe a research method that compares a process or outcome with a predetermined objective or with a control group. Audit is used to assess the extent to which an intervention meets a standard that is regarded as good practice. Monitoring is loosely synonymous with surveillance though the former term implies a more passive process of data collection and analysis than the latter. The results of this step are then used to inform steps 1 and 2 in a feedback loop. The three steps could therefore be viewed as an iterative, circular series of stepping stones rather than as a stepladder.

Screening or early disease detection (a type of secondary prevention) has been subjected to a rather specialised form of evaluation that takes account of its peculiar ethical imperatives. The principles or criteria for screening were first enumerated by Wilson and Jungner (1968) and subsequently updated by various authorities (including the UK National Screening Committee) and will not be elaborated in detail here. Their purpose was twofold: to ensure that the benefits and costs of a proposed screening programme were considered prior to implementation, and to provide a framework for evaluation once the screening programme had been running for a period of time. This example illustrates the way in which evaluation can straddle the time scale of an intervention rather than simply acting as a retrospective review of its successes and failures after the event.

Evaluation is sometimes dismissed as a dry, academic pursuit. In reality, it is a pragmatic, practical, problem-oriented and often highly creative activity. It is of such paramount importance, and so potentially contentious, that we will return to it at several points throughout this book, particularly in Chapters 6 and 12.

There is much more to public health, of course, than the concepts and methods outlined above but they offer a useful framework for addressing global public health in a systematic way. Although the three steps – diagnosis, treatment and follow-up – may appear to employ the language of clinical practice, they do not imply what some may regard as a reductionist 'medical model' of public health. On the contrary, the philosophy of this book is firmly anchored to inclusive, holistic and upstream modes of thinking rather than to a mechanistic biological one. The steps are intended to describe a logical, sequential theoretical framework for the entire gamut of public health activities and to depict public health in active, problem-solving 'response mode'. They also provide this book with its basic structure.

REFERENCES

Antonovsky A. *Health, Stress and Coping*. San Francisco: Jossey-Bass; 1979.

Department of Health. *Public Health in England: the report of the Committee of Inquiry into the Future Development of the Public Health Function (Acheson Report)*. London: HMSO; 1988.

Koplan JP, Bond TC, Merson MH, *et al.* Towards a common definition of global health. *Lancet*. 2009; **373**: 1993–5.

Lalonde M. *A New Perspective on the Health of Canadians*. Ottawa: National Health and Welfare; 1974.

McMichael A, Beaglehole R. The global context for public health. In: Beaglehole R, Bonita R, editors. *Global Public Health: a new era*. Oxford: Oxford University Press; 2009.

Minkler M. Health education, health promotion and the open society: an historical perspective. *Health Educ Q*. 1989; **16**(1): 17–30.

Sharma M, Atri A. *Essentials of International Health*. Sudbury, MA: Jones and Bartlett; 2010.

Skills for Health. *Functional Map of Public Health Practice*. Bristol: Skills for Health; 2002.

Wilson JMG, Jungner G. *Principles and Practice of Screening for Disease*. Geneva: World Health Organization; 1968.

World Health Organization. Constitution of the World Health Organization. *Chron World Health Organ*. 1974; **1**: 29–43.

World Health Organization. *Alma-Ata. Primary Health Care* (Health for All Series No. 1). Geneva: World Health Organization; 1978.

World Health Organization. *Ottawa Charter for Health Promotion*. Geneva: World Health Organization; 1986.

SECTION 1
Diagnosis

CHAPTER 1

The problem confronting humanity: an overview

The underlying premise (or, more accurately, hypothesis) of this book is that the world is facing (or is about to face) a major and potentially disastrous public health crisis that is all the more dangerous for its near invisibility. The purpose of this opening chapter is to state the case, in broad terms that encompass health as a whole, for that apparently hyperbolic assertion and to persuade the reader that the crisis is real – or at least imminent – and merits an urgent, vigorous response. Subsequent chapters examine some of the evidence for this assertion in greater detail.

I start by citing examples of the increasingly strident expressions of alarm about global health and then move on to examine whether or not this pessimism is justified. Following a review of some of the key concepts that epidemiologists use to 'diagnose' and describe health and disease in the population, I present demographic, mortality, morbidity and other data from a variety of sources in an attempt to offer the reader a reasonably comprehensive account of the current state of global health, highlighting especially the striking changes that have taken place (and are continuing to do so) in the global burden of disease over time. That is followed by a brief overview of the adverse public health consequences of past failures to act decisively and effectively.

The current state of global health is highly complex and cannot be easily summarised without oversimplification. Yet the effort is worthwhile if we are serious about understanding, and responding to, the public health challenge facing humanity in the early 21st century.

THE NEW PESSIMISM ABOUT GLOBAL HEALTH

> Today it has become almost a truism to call our time an age of anxiety.
> (Paul Tillich)

What is the cause of the relatively recent resurgence of concern about the state of global health and is it justified? Is it a manifestation of a growing awareness of our international interconnectedness and the need for a global perspective on health, a kind of byproduct of the broader phenomenon of globalisation? Are we simply responding to the previously poorly disseminated epidemiological evidence, and particularly the efforts of the World Health Organization (WHO) to raise the profile of health through the Global Burden of Disease (GBD) study? Have we been too complacent in the past and are we now paying a heavy price for our negligence? Has the seriousness of the alleged global health crisis been greatly exaggerated? Or are we simply over-reacting to dramatic media reporting of the ubiquitous presence of death and disease across the world, a state of affairs that has existed throughout history?

Those of us who are fortunate enough to live in affluent countries cannot help noticing the emergence, over the last 20 years or so, of a remarkably depressed discourse about the state of the world in general. We seem to be entering a new age of anxiety and discontent with our collective lot. Some of this negativity doubtless has specific triggers, such as fear of economic recession, climate change, peak oil, scarce water resources, demographic imbalances, terrorism, war or the appearance of new pandemics. For many, however, the malaise is general and reflects a vague sense of unease about a raft of fashionable grievances including the globalised market economy, Western political hegemony, corporate greed, environmental degradation, neocolonialism and large-scale abuses of human rights. All of this amounts to a protracted sense of disillusionment with modernity, however that is defined, that has its roots in the socioeconomic environment but impinges harshly on the individual psyche. Wilkinson and Pickett (2010) articulate this well in the opening chapter of their book *The Spirit Level*.

> It is a remarkable paradox that, at the pinnacle of human material and technical achievement, we find ourselves anxiety-ridden, prone to depression, worried about how others see us, unsure of our friendships, driven to consume and with little or no community life. Lacking the relaxed social contact and emotional satisfaction we all need, we seek comfort in overeating, obsessive shopping and spending, or become prey to excessive alcohol, psychoactive medicines and illegal drugs. (p.93) (Reproduced by permission of Penguin Books Ltd)

This is not an evidence-based statement but rather a heartfelt expression of collective social pain. The writers go on to develop this theme into a full-blown hypothesis that might explain, via psychosocial pathways, the clear statistical correlation between income inequality and poor health. But is this bleak description of contemporary life actually true? Or does it merely represent a jaundiced worldview, rooted in a nostalgic yearning for past ideological certainties, that has again become prevalent among sectors of the English-speaking middle classes? We can't answer those questions with confidence but there does seem to be a *zeitgeist* of gloom afoot in some Western countries that may be contributing to a general sense of unhappiness and foreboding.

Here is another example from New Zealand-based academics writing at the end of the 20th century. Beaglehole and Bonita (1997) adopt a more macroeconomic perspective on contemporary public health. Their broadside focuses on the allegedly stifling impact of neoliberal economic policies on global health, combined with an attack on individualism and the alleged indifference of the modern consumer society to the environment. Their critique seems predicated, perhaps deliberately, on an unmistakeably left-of-centre worldview.

> The 'new world order' of the 1990s is, in general, not conducive to public health. The global economy is increasingly integrated under the banner of 'free trade' and 'market forces.' ... The dominance of the ideology of individualism causes serious difficulties for the collective actions which are at the core of effective public health policy and programmes. The response to widespread environmental damage has so far been minimal. Our vulnerability to disease could readily be exposed by subtle environmental changes or a breakdown in basic public health services. (p.230) (Reproduced by permission of Cambridge University Press)

Wolinsky (2000) goes even further and warns that we are all, including the developed world, sleepwalking towards disaster. He argues that, notwithstanding advances in modern medicine, the people of the industrialised world are completely unprepared for the profound challenges of what he foresees as an impending and large-scale public health catastrophe.

Raziz (2010) sees no glimmer of light a decade later.

> The human prospect is uncertain. The social and ecological crisis is deep and prolonged and is a historic crisis for it calls the basic premises, the basic presupposition upon which our culture is based, into question. (p.473)

Using graphic and sometimes violent imagery, Roberts (2011) links obesity, climate change and fossil fuels into a single toxic environmental knot that threatens to strangle humanity. Arguing that greenhouse gases threaten 'generational genocide' and that petroleum is 'the lethal kinetic energy that bullies people from the streets and into their cars', he seems to see the dark arts of 'fossil fuel industry propaganda' as a major (if not the main) cause of hunger, war, obesity and ill health as well as environmental damage.

Readers will doubtless have encountered many other examples of this kind of doom-laden prognostication from otherwise sober and thoughtful writers.

Are they suffering from a collective, millenarian neurosis or even delusion? Or could they be right? Much of the rest of this book will be devoted to trying to answer those questions.

Is the recent economic downturn the problem?

In considering the various factors that are invoked to explain the prevailing gloomy atmosphere in which discussion on public health often seems shrouded, we should not underestimate one particularly corrosive influence. Perhaps, to quote President Bill Clinton (in another context), 'it's the economy, stupid'. As the world counts the cost of the recent economic recession and struggles to reduce public expenditure, the health sector has found itself caught up in this predicament, to its extreme discomfiture. The UK National Health Service, for example, is currently on the receiving end of attention of a kind that is potentially threatening. Indeed, it may be nearing the end of an era of unprecedented financial investment and organisational expansion. Efficiency drives and other forms of managerial intrusion are placing great strain on all who work within it and demoralisation is widespread. The public health community, much of which is closely dependent on the NHS, is not immune to such processes.

Not that the impact of economic factors on health is purely organisational, important though that undoubtedly is. Nor should they be regarded as purely subjective irritants of the 'healthcare commentariat' that alter our perceptions rather than reality. We know, from decades of epidemiological research, that there is a close statistical correlation between health and wealth and that the global economic downturn will, sooner or later, adversely impinge on health as measured by reported rates of mortality, morbidity and wellbeing in most countries (Stuckler *et al* 2009). The new global health crisis could arguably simply reflect the new global economic crisis. Superficially, that may be an appealing explanation but it doesn't hold water. All the evidence suggests that the global economic downturn that started in 2008 was an exacerbating rather than causal factor. The global public health crisis has been brewing for at least two decades and probably much longer. Where the global economic crisis has perhaps inflicted the greatest damage has been to demoralise all those, including Sir Michael Marmot, who have argued that social inequalities in health were remediable within a generation (Commission on Social Determinants of Health 2008). That now seems a wildly optimistic scenario, comparable in its naivety to the Health for All by the Year 2000 objective proclaimed by the WHO at Alma-Ata (World Health Organization 1978).

Nevertheless, a recurring theme in discussions around global health is the close link between poverty and ill health. The poorest countries tend to have the worst health outcomes, and poor health inhibits economic productivity. There is thus a strong mutual interdependence between global public health and the global economy. Professional economists increasingly regard public health as a key precondition for successful economic development (Sachs 2005). We shall explore some of the reasons for this later in the book.

Energy, the environment and the global crisis

Homer-Dixon (2006) contends that five 'tectonic stresses' are building inexorably beneath the surface of today's global order:

➤ energy stress, especially from increasing scarcity of conventional oil
➤ economic stress from greater global economic instability and widening income gaps between rich and poor
➤ demographic stress from differentials in population growth rates between rich and poor societies and from expansion of megacities in poor societies
➤ environmental stress from worsening damage to land, water, forests and fisheries
➤ climate stress from changes in the composition of the earth's atmosphere.

Of these, energy stress is of paramount importance because energy is humanity's master resource. When energy is scarce and costly, it adversely affects all human activity including economic growth, food and water production, information exchange and defence. The effect of the five stresses is magnified by increasing international connectivity and by the escalating power of small extremist groups to destroy infrastructure and people, including, potentially, entire cities. These stresses and multipliers combine into a potentially lethal mixture. Together, they greatly increase the risk of a cascading collapse of systems vital to our wellbeing, a phenomenon Homer-Dixon calls 'synchronous failure'. Societies must do everything they can to avoid such an outcome. The challenges we face today are comparable, he argues, to those faced by the Roman Empire almost 2000 years ago.

Homer-Dixon is not entirely pessimistic. There are solutions, he assures us. If people are well prepared, they may be able to exploit less extreme forms of breakdown to achieve radical reform and the renewal of institutions, social relations, technologies, and entrenched forms of destructive behaviour. Homer-Dixon sees most of these threats as opportunities.

These quasi-political reflections on the current state of global health draw, in part at least, on an interpretation of the available information. Our first priority is to seek an answer to what appears at first sight to be a simple question. What is the state of health of the world's population? In answering it, we must briefly examine the way that population health is measured, analysed and interpreted by epidemiologists.

INDICATORS OF GLOBAL PUBLIC HEALTH

If we employ the metaphor, alluded to earlier, of the world's population as our patient, what are the 'symptoms and signs' of ill health, what is the public health 'diagnosis' on which interventions ('treatment') should be based, and why should we regard any of this as relevant to our understanding of the global health crisis confronting humanity at the outset of the 21st century?

Just as a doctor assesses the state of health of an individual patient by means of a set of well-established methods (taking a history, performing a clinical examination, undertaking laboratory tests), a public health professional assesses the state of health of a population – any population – using epidemiological techniques. Epidemiology, the basic science of public health, has evolved rapidly over the past 150 years. Its methods have become increasingly systematic, standardised and reliable. To understand the state of global health, we need to have some insight into the nature and *modus operandi* of epidemiology.

Epidemiology is a branch of medical or biological science that may be defined as: 'the study of the distribution and determinants of health and disease in human populations'. By 'distribution' is meant the frequency of occurrence of health and disease in the population as a whole or within specified sub-groups, while 'determinants' simply means causes or influences (such as risk factors). For our present purposes, the 'distribution of health and disease' is the important part of this definition. It refers to *descriptive epidemiology* rather than analytical or evaluational techniques, though there is some overlap between them. And descriptive epidemiology has proven itself to be an extremely powerful tool for characterising the state of population health.

Epidemiologists – or at least those involved in this particular field of public health activity (known as descriptive epidemiology or needs assessment) – use a range of quantitative indicators (such as incidence and prevalence) to assess and describe the state of health of a population, either as a whole or (more usually) in terms of its constituent parts. Widely used indicators of population health are derived from demographic, mortality, morbidity (including disability), healthcare utilisation and survey data. Much of this information is accessible, to a greater or lesser extent, via routinely collected and published statistics in high-income countries and to a much lesser extent in low- and medium-income countries. All the indicators have their particular methodological strengths and weaknesses, and these often vary from country to country and region to region. As in clinical medicine, the process of arriving at an epidemiological diagnosis is not a scientifically precise activity, and relies on the exercise of a degree of judgement that is open to challenge.

Demography

Because epidemiology is a population-based science, it depends, above all, on the existence of detailed knowledge both about the numbers and characteristics of people who suffer from diseases or disorders – the *numerators* – and about the population at risk – the *denominators*. Denominators, in turn, are derived in large part from total population estimates, usually calculated from projections and assumptions based on periodic population censuses, adjusted for births, deaths and (where possible) migration, provided by national statistical agencies. Adequate information about the numbers of births and deaths in a particular country or region is necessary for these calculations to have any validity. That information is often lacking or extremely unreliable. Even the most basic information about the estimated size of a population at a given time may be non-existent. Some researchers have estimated that more than a third of the world's 128 million annual births are not registered (Setel *et al* 2007).

Once denominators are available – and that scenario can never be taken for granted – they may be used for three main purposes. First, demographic statistics tell us much about the health of a population, notably its stability, its fertility and its age–sex structure. Second, demographers use these statistics to project population growth into the future, thereby enabling governments to plan services that will meet the needs of countries, regions and communities. Third, populations or groups can be compared with respect to the rates or proportions that suffer from particular disorders or risk factors. All of these characteristics are important in assessing population health.

Mortality, morbidity and disability

Disease affects all populations in ways that are remarkably consistent. Malnutrition and infection have (at least until recently) been the dominant threats to health in the poorest countries while cancer, cardiovascular and other chronic diseases are the headline grabbers in the richest; mental illness and trauma afflict all communities. Nevertheless, there are outliers, countries that buck the trend in terms of unexpectedly high or low death or occurrence (incidence and prevalence) rates from certain diseases. Epidemiologists describe these patterns and variations – though they don't always succeed in explaining them – in terms of mortality (death rates) and morbidity (ill health rates) in the population. Disability – chronic ill health that interferes with daily living – is especially important in assessing the impact of a disease on quality of life and may affect up to 15% of the world's population (World Health Organization/World Bank 2011). Accurate data on this neglected health dimension are rarely collected, thereby severely hampering national and international efforts to identify and meet the needs of disabled people. Data on disability are sometimes subsumed under the morbidity heading and are increasingly incorporated into the assessment of the burden of disease on a population (*see* Chapter 2).

A helpful way to think of the epidemiology of any condition is to visualise an iceberg or pyramid with mortality at the tip, hospitalisations in the middle and incidence, including premorbid and with causal or risk factors, at the base. It must be remembered that (mainly at or near the base of the pyramid) large numbers of patients present to health services in ways that are not captured at all by routine statistics. Illness in children, especially, may be self-treated or managed by parents or carers or by community practitioners such as nurses, family doctors or teachers. Only some of these incidents will be recorded and those that are may not be easily accessible. A widely held assumption is that most severe illnesses will be treated initially in hospital emergency departments (EDs), where these facilities are available. Even then, data from EDs are extremely patchy due to variations in recording or reporting practice and the lack of clearly defined catchment areas, rendering denominators almost impossible to quantify. Ideally, all EDs would record and report such information but this is rarely undertaken.

An example of the epidemiological pyramid is one that is often used to describe injury (Figure 1.1), showing mortality in the upper section, morbidity (manifested as disability and injuries) in the middle, and antecedents (risk factors, precursors and preinjury incidents) at the base. The pyramid is conceptual rather than an accurate representation of the numerical scale of each layer. Nevertheless, it is a salutary reminder of the relatively small proportion of all injuries that result in death. Near the base of the pyramid lie the very large number of incidents (such as falls, road crashes) that may or may not cause an injury, or that lead to relatively trivial bumps, scrapes, sprains and other outcomes that require no attention from a healthcare professional. And at the base are the even more numerous antecedent events (such as discarding of lighted cigarettes, cycling without a helmet) that place individuals at increased risk of an incident that could cause an injury. From a public health perspective, all the layers are important both in assessing the scale of the challenge and in planning countermeasures.

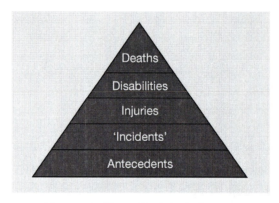

Figure 1.1 The epidemiological pyramid.

As well as illustrating graphically the relative numerical importance of the various levels of severity of a disease or disorder, the pyramid metaphor has an additional value. It can help us elucidate aetiology in specific diseases as well as merely describing the state of population health. That is because the layers are connected to each other in an approximately sequential manner. By rotating the pyramid through 90°, it becomes transformed into a sequence of successive and inter-related events or a 'natural history of disease' that starts with suscepti-bility or exposure to risk factors, leads to physiological (or psychological) dys-function and established disease, and culminates in either an adverse outcome (such death or disability) or resolution. That enhanced understanding of the disease process may, in turn, be used to stimulate thinking about prevention or at least control. Once the natural history of any disease process is understood, it becomes possible to develop, implement and evaluate strategies to arrest or reverse the process and thereby reduce the number of victims, the impact of the disorder and the burden of the condition on the population at risk.

Routine mortality data

Although mortality occupies only the tip of the disease pyramid, it is the most extensively studied for various reasons. Death, unlike illness, is (usually) an unambiguous and unequivocal event. It is also widely regarded as the most serious outcome of a disease, is well understood by non-professionals and thus has particular public health importance. The reporting of *mortality statistics* is a statutory requirement in most countries of the world although in practice, their completeness and quality vary widely. It is hugely tempting to accept disease mortality rates at their face value but this would be a mistake. They are liable to contain numerous sources of error, including incompleteness, diagnostic inac-curacy, misclassification and bias, as these are almost inevitable in the produc-tion of such statistics. Because the quality of mortality data is so inconsistent between countries, international comparisons present major problems.

Setel *et al* (2007) highlight the depressing fact that fewer than a third of the nearly 60 million deaths in the world each year are medically certified or registered. Under-reporting is especially prevalent in the countries of Africa and Asia with the poorest health (Figure 1.2; *see* colour plate section between pages 46 and 47). Estimates of mortality and disease burden are therefore often dependent on extrapolations from relatively small and unreliable household surveys. Moreover, mortality is the outcome of an interaction between disease incidence, severity and survival, each of which is influenced by a multiplicity of factors. Even where death is registered, its cause may be unknown or a matter of speculation based on, at best, a postmortem or accounts offered by relatives or other carers ('verbal autopsy'). Nevertheless, mortality data have always been attractive to epidemiologists because of their far greater availability and acces-sibility than other indicators.

Routine morbidity data

Morbidity is variously defined either as a state of departure from physical or mental health or, when expressed by epidemiologists as a rate, as the incidence or prevalence of disease in the population. It occupies the middle region of the pyramid and is much more important numerically in a population than mortality. Because we all suffer from illness several times in our lives but only die once, morbidity is arguably a much better indicator of the overall state of health of a population, and its quality of life, than mortality. Morbidity and disability data are, however, seldom prioritised or reported by national statistical agencies because they require relatively sophisticated and expensive epidemiological techniques, such as validated questionnaires distributed to representative samples of the population, to generate them.

Specific forms of morbidity may be reported by specially constructed data collection systems maintained within national or local information offices that are generally designed to support health protection. These monitoring or surveillance systems include databases (sometimes called registers or registries) on cancer, diabetes, infectious diseases, trauma and birth defects. All have their peculiar advantages and disadvantages, depending on circumstances, and the balance between the two may change over time. They help to plug the information gap at the centre of the disease pyramid and provide unrivalled insights into the epidemiology of disorders that would otherwise be neglected or subjected to uninformed speculation. At their best, they have proved invaluable sources of data for research, to monitor trends, to identify epidemics and clusters, and to introduce preventive or therapeutic countermeasures. On the other hand, they are resource intensive and bureaucratic. And growing concerns about data confidentiality, consent and the ethical or legal context have begun to cast a shadow over the operation of many of these databases in recent years. They are almost entirely confined to affluent countries.

Health surveys

Periodic population health surveys offer alternative and, to epidemiologists, extremely valuable sources of information about the state of health, including the prevalence of disease and disability, of a population. Examples of such surveys in the UK include the decennial Census, the General Household Survey, the Scottish and English Health Surveys (of adults) and long-term research studies (e.g. the Avon Longitudinal Study of Parents and Children, the Millennium Cohort Study) conducted by academic departments for specific purposes. There are similar surveys in North America, including the US National Health and Nutrition Examination Study (of adults and children), mainland Europe and in several other parts of the world. If conducted properly, they are the most detailed and reliable sources of information on disease incidence and prevalence. Virtually all the other indicators of population health are second-hand in that they depend on the occurrence and reporting of subsequent events, such as death or hospital admission, rather than on the illness itself. Clinicians, administrators or relatives often report these secondary events through the filter of bureaucratic systems that may or may not accurately reflect either the occurrence or the nature of the disease or disorder. *Ad hoc* or periodic surveys have further advantages over routine vital or healthcare statistics in that they are not so supply dependent; a community without dentists, for example, may appear to have no dental caries even when many people suffer from the condition. Nevertheless, surveys are subject to the usual sources of epidemiological error including artefact, bias, confounding and chance.

Healthcare usage

In the absence of accurate morbidity data derived from surveys, other sources of information about the state of population health are worth considering. One of these is the number and nature of contacts that patients make with healthcare facilities. Because of their expense, healthcare systems, at least in developed countries, are usually subjected to detailed accounting and audit processes that involve monitoring of the numbers of people using services along with some demographic and diagnostic or procedural data. This type of information can be helpful to epidemiologists as well as managers as it generates data on healthcare utilisation – hospital admissions, ED and outpatient visits, etc. – that may be used to monitor, albeit crudely, population health (or, more accurately, ill health) beyond mortality statistics.

Unfortunately, there are several serious drawbacks to using healthcare utilisation data for epidemiological purposes. At first sight, healthcare statistics fit the bill as proxy indicators of ill health. It seems logical to assume that people who are ill will make use of health services where they are provided. With a moment's reflection, however, serious flaws in this argument become apparent. First, not all sick people present to health services for a variety of reasons including geographical barriers, cost, inconvenience, ignorance and fear. Second, some people present inappropriately with anxieties (the 'worried well') or even entrenched delusions about the presence of non-existent illness. And third, the very existence of a healthcare facility, such as a dental surgery or a new local hospital, will generate demand while its absence will diminish it.

Hospitalisation statistics are particularly problematic. Not only are they subject to the same sources of error as mortality data, they suffer from the added disadvantage of being dependent to a large extent on the local availability and deployment of hospital beds. To add to the confusion, hospital admission policies for the same condition may vary widely between hospitals and that will distort the data patterns. Thus a low hospitalisation rate may reflect a low level of bed provision or a tendency not to admit patients, rather than a low incidence of disease. Furthermore, the completeness and accuracy of the diagnostic coding of hospitalisation data may vary widely between hospitals, communities and countries. We cannot escape the conclusion that data based on healthcare contacts represent an extremely unsatisfactory measure of population health. They are extensively used for epidemiological purposes because, like mortality statistics, they are available in many countries due to their cost implications for service providers or governments. And one stark fact stands out from all the others – healthcare costs are rising exponentially around the world, especially in high-income countries. That is one of the major motivating factors for governments to support public health initiatives on the grounds that prevention is presumed (sometimes wrongly) to be cheaper, as well as more desirable, than cure.

To sum up this overview of epidemiological indicators: mortality (death) statistics tend to be more frequently cited by epidemiologists than morbidity (illness and disability) estimates simply because they are more often available. Both have their place in descriptive epidemiology, as do several other indicators, such as registries and periodic surveys of health and wellbeing. Healthcare utilisation statistics are probably the least satisfactory form of information about population health.

THE CURRENT STATUS OF GLOBAL POPULATION HEALTH: A THUMBNAIL SKETCH

In very broad-brush terms, we can use demographic, mortality, morbidity and healthcare statistics, where they exist, to attempt to describe the current health of the world's population. What do these epidemiological indicators tell us about the state of global health? The next chapter tries to provide a detailed answer but here are the headlines.

➤ The main threat arising from demography has been the sheer numbers of people inhabiting the planet. The current population of the earth has rocketed in the last two centuries from around 900 million in 1800 to around 7 billion today. This is expected to rise to around 9 billion by 2050, thereafter flattening out. Clearly there must be a limit to the total population that can be safely and healthily sustained by available resources, particularly in the context of the stresses produced by dwindling reserves of oil and water, climate change and repeated economic downturns. Other demographic trends, such as falling fertility and a rising proportion of elderly people, are also potentially deleterious to health (*see* the demographic transition, Chapter 2).

➤ Mortality rates have been declining steadily, from all and specific causes, in most countries of the world over the last 200 years. Some of these improvements may be attributed to demographic, social, environmental or economic factors while others are due to deliberate environmental, legislative or healthcare interventions. Many are totally or partially unexplained. Yet the bottom line is that falling infant and child mortality rates, combined with steady nutritional and environmental improvements, have prolonged life expectancy and enhanced the quality of life for most of the earth's population.

➤ The world still faces a long list of health challenges: persistent social, ethnic, gender and geographical inequalities in health, and a growing burden of chronic disease (much of which is attributable to tobacco and alcohol), unintentional injuries, infections such as HIV/AIDS, malaria and tuberculosis (TB), malnutrition, obesity, disability and mental illness. To these conventional health threats may be added more recent fears of the health impact of climate change, environmental damage, civil unrest, human rights abuses, interpersonal violence, terrorism and armed conflict.

➤ All diseases and causes of premature death disproportionately affect poorer communities; 90% of the roughly 59 million deaths worldwide each year occur in low- and middle-income countries. Both mortality and morbidity rates vary enormously between and within countries in relation to age, gender, ethnicity, geography and time. Mortality rates have tended to decline more rapidly in high- and medium-income countries than in low-income countries, in part due to varying rates of economic and infrastructural development including environmental engineering and healthcare initiatives. That divergence has exacerbated pre-existing health inequalities between countries and regions.

➤ Estimating the national and global burden of disease and disability remains severely hampered by the inadequacy of available information relating to all levels of the epidemiological pyramid, especially its middle and base. International and regional health comparisons, and time trends, should be subject to careful qualification due to the great variability in data completeness, quality, accessibility, classification and reporting, quite apart from the difficulty in interpreting the reasons for any variations identified in this way.

These are largely unsurprising and uncontroversial generalisations about the state of global health. And like all generalisations, what they conceal may be more important than what they reveal. Diseases, disorders and risks that are not properly recorded and reported will remain inadequately enumerated, investigated and prevented. A recurring theme of this book is the serious paucity of relevant and accurate epidemiological information about common diseases and their impact. Such data are essential to enable us to undertake the kinds of detailed investigation necessary to document and explain health trends in time and place, both nationally and internationally. Data are, of course, merely an epidemiological means to a public health end. But if the means is seriously flawed, the end is unlikely to be achieved.

DETERMINANTS OF HEALTH

Once we have performed a 'needs assessment' on the state of global health, the next task is to seek to understand the underlying reasons for the varying patterns of health and disease that we observe around the world. That understanding should, in turn, help us to intervene more effectively to prevent disease and improve health. We should recognise the formidable nature of this task: disease causation and health promotion are highly complex processes that remain only partially explained. Following the large-scale environmental and engineering programmes, combined with advances in the biological sciences and the introduction of state-funded public services of the 19th century, much epidemiological attention was paid in the 20th century to the identification and control of risk factors such as smoking and diet. All these approaches achieved undeniably impressive results in the past and doubtless will continue to play a role in the future. There is a widespread feeling, however, that new theoretical paradigms, particularly about the causation of ill health, are required if we are to maintain the momentum of global health improvement into the 21st century.

Although every disorder has its own specific causal process or natural history, attempts have been made to generalise about the key determinants of population health. Canadian writers have provided us with some useful insights. A Minister of Health, Lalonde (1974), coined the phrase the 'health field concept' (Box 1.1) that looked deceptively simple yet paved the way for more sophisticated thinking. The health field, he wrote, comprises four ele-

---

BOX 1.1 *Lalonde's health field concept*

➤ *Environment*
All influences on health outside the human body and over which the individual has little or no control. Includes the physical and social environment.
➤ *Human Biology*
All aspects of health, physical and mental, developed within the human body as a result of organic make-up.
➤ *Lifestyle*
The aggregation of personal decisions, over which the individual has control. Self-imposed risks created by unhealthy lifestyle choices can be said to contribute to, or cause, illness or death.
➤ *Healthcare Organisation*
The quantity, quality, arrangement, nature and relationships of people and resources in the provision of healthcare.

ments: biology, lifestyle, environment and health services. This model proved especially helpful in focusing the minds of public health policy makers on factors other than human behaviour. Its great strength was to refocus attention on both the environment and healthcare as key influences on health. Much public health strategic thinking at that time had become bogged down in a rather narrow view of health promotion that appeared excessively preoccupied with educating people to change their behaviour in a more health-enhancing direction. The health field concept placed behaviour in the context of other health determinants that, according to Lalonde, were equally or more important than lifestyle, risk taking and other types of individual decision making.

Lalonde expressed contemporary ideas about health determinants in a succinct and intuitively plausible manner. It was rare, at that time, for a government ministry to acknowledge the multifactorial nature of health and disease and to commit itself to pursuing population health improvement in ways that moved beyond exhortations to individuals to change their health-destructive lifestyles.

Public health experts and agencies found the model an exceptionally powerful tool for analysing and advocating a holistic approach to addressing health challenges. They soon discovered, however, that the public health planning process strained the Lalonde model close to breaking point. The Canadian government subsequently expanded it to include additional factors such as social capital, culture, education and literacy, child development and employment. They also split the environment into physical and social components. Others embellished the concept in various ways in an attempt to introduce a

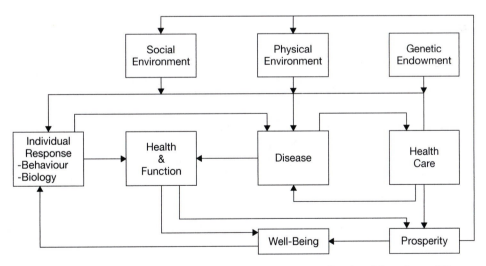

Figure 1.3 Evans and Stoddart model of health promotion. Reprinted from Evans RG, Stoddart GL. Producing health, consuming health care. *Soc Sci Med.* 1990; **31**: 1347–63, with permission from Elsevier.

greater degree of both complexity and specificity. A notable expression of this development was the attempt by Evans and Stoddart (1990) to identify the links between the various factors influencing health outcomes (Fig. 1.3). Their insights may be summed up by the phrase 'everything matters'.

A key problem with this multidimensional, causal loop approach is that its all-encompassing scope can induce confusion. As the UK government discovered, when applied to highly complex public health challenges, such as obesity (Foresight 2007), the ensuing proliferation of boxes and multidirectional arrows is liable to be virtually indecipherable to most general readers and thus potentially counterproductive.

In an attempt to restore a sense of conceptual coherence to these theories, Dahlgren and Whitehead (1991) proposed a 'rainbow' comprising a series of concentric circles around the individual at the core. Their concept encompassed a wide range of environmental determinants of health along with those operating at community, social and individual level (Figure 1.4). This model retained some of the simplicity of Lalonde's health field concept while introducing some additional subtler elements such as social networks, occupational factors and general socioeconomic conditions. While emphasising the connectivity between the various groups of variables, Dahlgren and Whitehead may perhaps have neglected some important contextual factors, such as cultural practices and interpersonal relationships, which tend to transcend many of the specific components.

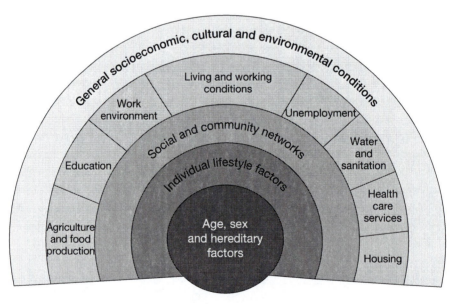

Figure 1.4 Dahlgren and Whitehead model of health determinants. Source: Dahlgren G, Whitehead M. *Policies and Strategies to Promote Social Equity in Health.* Stockholm: Institute of Futures Studies; 1991. www.framtidsstudier.se

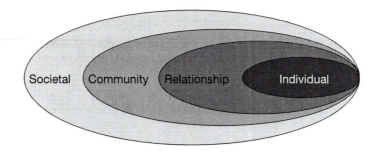

Figure 1.5 Dahlberg and Krug's Social Ecological Model. Source: Dahlberg LL, Krug EG. Violence – a global public health problem. In: Krug E, Dahlberg LL, Mercy JA, *et al*, editors. *World Report on Violence and Health*. Geneva: World Health Organization; 2002. pp.1–56.

A variant of the 'rainbow' is the Social Ecological Model (Figure 1.5) proposed by Dahlberg and Krug (2002). It has been highly influential in the evolving thinking around the prevention of injury and violence of both the USA Centers for Disease Control and the WHO though it is equally applicable to many other aspects of health. This model represents the complex interplay between individual, relationship, community and societal factors that put people at risk. Like the rainbow model, the individual sits at the centre of an overlapping series of concentric circles. Its practical implication is that preventive strategies should include developmentally appropriate activities addressing multiple levels of the model, all of which impinge, to a greater or lesser extent, on individuals to varying degrees across the lifespan.

Individual
The first level focuses on biological and personal factors that increase the risk of disease or injury. Examples include age, education, income, personality, illness and history of substance abuse.

Relationship
The second level includes factors that increase risk through human relationships of all kinds – with parents, siblings, peers, intimate partners and others. These relationships influence behaviour and contribute to exposure to risk.

Community
The third level encompasses the various settings (e.g. schools, workplaces, neighbourhoods) in which relationships occur and attempts to identify the characteristics of these settings that influence risk.

Societal
The fourth level addresses the broad societal factors that provide a context within which a disease is more or less likely to occur. These factors include

social and cultural norms, government policies and macroeconomic processes that influence social inequalities in the population.

More theories of health

In parallel with the development of these theories, epidemiologists and social scientists were undertaking empirical research that led to further speculation around the underlying determinants of health. Some of these focused on socioeconomic factors and the production of health inequalities, others on biological, psychological and social influences or 'programming' at sensitive points during the human lifecycle. Those approaches are discussed in detail later in this book.

A third cluster of researchers has been investigating the profound implications of a hypothesis that had its origins in the study of Holocaust survivors living in Israel. Antonovsky (1979) posed the question: what creates health? His starting point was the observation that some people seem more resilient than others to stresses and risks, sometimes of an extreme nature, that would normally be expected to damage health. He postulated that health-promoting or 'salutogenic' processes are dependent on two sets of individual characteristics: 'resistance' factors (such as identity and social support) and the 'sense of coherence' (SOC), a measure of the extent to which people make sense of their experiences and environment. These characteristics are primarily acquired early in childhood as a result of a nurturing family life combined with adequate material resources along with a supportive social and cultural context. Several studies around the world have demonstrated positive correlations between the SOC and perceived health (especially mental health) and quality of life. Eriksson and Lindstrom (2008) have urged the health promotion community to integrate Antonovsky's ideas with the lifecourse approach in a way that reinforces the goals of the Ottawa Charter (*see* Chapter 7).

We will return to the theme of health determinants throughout the book. It is impossible to intervene effectively in public health by focusing exclusively on outcomes without paying heed to the causal chains that lead to them.

CRISIS? WHAT CRISIS?

A legitimate question before we proceed further is this: if global public health is in a state of crisis, albeit barely recognised, where is the evidence? After all, enormous advances have been made in nutrition, environmental hygiene, immunisations, road safety, healthcare and a multiplicity of other areas over the past 150 years. These have benefited all people in all parts of the world. In wealthy countries, neonatal care, cancer therapy and coronary bypass surgery are three fields that have improved survival in patients almost beyond recognition over the past few decades. Both preventive and therapeutic interventions, including drugs and sophisticated healthcare technologies, are being rapidly disseminated to poorer countries. This is reflected in improving life expectancy in most parts of the world. If the global population is our patient, isn't he in rather rude health and getting progressively healthier with every passing year? The answer is yes and no, as Chapter 2 will illustrate.

The word 'crisis' suggests a peak of danger or a decisive turning point at a particular point in time. We perceive the crisis when events, observed longitudinally, take a turn for the worse and the turning point may only be recognised retrospectively. Moreover, the process may be prolonged; a crisis arising acutely may become chronic if it doesn't resolve. The diagnosis of a crisis must be made in the context of a particular time frame. For our purpose, the turn of the millennium is as good a starting point as any.

By 1999, there was undeniable evidence of improving global health (Garrett 2000); life expectancies were soaring across the globe, in both affluent industrialised countries and in many poorer countries as well. The World Health Organization forecast that average life expectancy globally would reach 73 years by 2025, up from only 48 in 1955. Moreover, the number of child deaths before the age of five had plummeted from 21 million in 1955 to 11 million in 1995.

A recent analysis (Kebede-Francis 2011) was even more upbeat, revealing that more than half of the world population was living longer and healthier and a third of the world population was making progress towards those ends.

At the same time, there was a worrying countercurrent. Despite promising overall trends, several simultaneous local and regional reversals were profoundly disturbing to health experts. The dual epidemics of TB and AIDS undermined sub-Saharan Africa's hard-won health advances, with life expectancies slumping alarmingly. Malawi's average life expectancy, for example, fell below its pre-World War II levels, due almost entirely to the human immunodeficiency virus.

As we shall see throughout this book, we are confronting a mixed picture containing both positive and negative elements. How we view it is, in part, highly subjective. Does this amount to a global public health crisis, either current or impending? Without being dogmatic about the answer, prudence dictates that we should tend towards the view that it does. This is one of those 'glass half full versus glass half empty' scenarios. Either way, we need to act to preserve the gains we have made. This is more difficult as the crisis (if it exists) has been a prolonged one, a slow-burn rather than a sudden explosion. Although the evidence is equivocal, most of the data suggest that the state of global health and wellbeing is likely to deteriorate further unless we take evasive action. While we may argue about terminology and time scales, there is little doubt that the global public health challenge is real – or at least imminent – rather than imaginary, and demands a response.

To avoid the balance of global health tipping towards an irreversible downward spiral, we should be able to recognise what clinicians call 'red light symptoms and signs'. One of these is the resurgence of many of the 'old' infectious diseases in all countries, but particularly the poorer ones. Other negative signs include rising maternal mortality, after decades of decline, in some developed countries, plummeting life expectancy in the former Soviet Union (notably in the period 1990–2000), new infectious agents (e.g. *Cryptosporidium* and *Legionella*), increasing microbial resistance to antibiotics, diminishing herd immunity, an ageing population, widening inequalities in health, crumbling public health infrastructures and escalating healthcare costs. All of these sources of concern are greatly magnified by the context of the simultaneous stresses arising from energy shortages, shifting demographic patterns, macroeconomic downturns, environmental disruption and climate change.

CONSEQUENCES OF PAST FAILURE TO ADDRESS GLOBAL HEALTH CHALLENGES

We will explore in greater detail in Chapter 5 some of the reasons for our failure to address global public health challenges more effectively. The result is that we now face extremely serious short- and long-term consequences: potentially avoidable mortality and morbidity, chronic anxiety about health, widespread human suffering and persistent health inequalities between and within countries. That list, partial as it is, would be depressing enough. If we add to it the looming environmental threats of global warming, the loss of biodiversity and inadequate natural resources to support the world's increasing population, we are facing a conglomeration of problems that, taken together, could pose a real if only dimly recognised risk to the future of *Homo sapiens*. That may seem an alarmist vision but it is one that has attracted a growing band of influential adherents.

Even if we reject the most extreme and apocalyptic scenarios, there is no denying the unacceptably low levels of health and wellbeing of large numbers of people on the planet, particularly in its poorer regions. Many of them have succumbed and will continue to succumb to life-threatening and avoidable disorders. Because of the circular relationship between socioeconomic factors and health (since poverty not only causes ill health but is, in turn, exacerbated by it), the prospects of reducing social inequalities in health are reduced, it seems, to near zero. Breaking the cycle will require determination and focus.

The European Commission has urged all countries to invest strongly in health in the light of the evidence that health is a driver of economic growth, especially in low-income countries (Suhrcke *et al* 2005). For the most affluent parts of the world, the longer term and subtler consequences of poor health are no less serious and socially corrosive. Among its more obvious effects are dramatically escalating healthcare costs, declining productivity, economic stagnation, persistent poverty, unfulfilled public expectations, professional demoralisation, widespread nihilism, a retreat to irrational and ineffective remedies such as homeopathy and a self-destructive tendency, especially among the young, to live for the present at the expense of the future.

REFERENCES

Antonovsky A. *Health, Stress and Coping*. San Francisco: Jossey-Bass; 1979.

Beaglehole R, Bonita R. *Public Health at the Crossroads: achievements and prospects*. Cambridge: Cambridge University Press; 1997.

Commission on Social Determinants of Health. *Closing the Gap in a Generation: health equity through action on the social determinants of health*. CSDH Final Report. Geneva: World Health Organization; 2008.

Dahlberg LL, Krug EG. Violence – a global public health problem. In: Krug E, Dahlberg LL, Mercy JA, *et al*, editors. *World Report on Violence and Health*. Geneva: World Health Organization; 2002. pp.1–56.

Dahlgren G, Whitehead M. *Policies and Strategies to Promote Social Equity in Health*. Stockholm: Institute of Futures Studies; 1991.

Eriksson M, Lindstrom B. A salutogenic interpretation of the Ottawa Charter. *Health Promot Int*. 2008; **23**: 190–9.

Evans RG, Stoddart GL. Producing health, consuming health care. *Soc Sci Med*. 1990; **31**: 1347–63.

Foresight. *Tackling Obesities: future choices – building the obesity system map*. London: Government Office for Science; 2007.

Garrett L. *Betrayal of Trust: the collapse of global public health*. New York: Hyperion; 2000.

Homer-Dixon T. *The Upside of Down. Catastrophe, creativity and the renewal of civilisation*. Toronto: Knopf; 2006.

Kebede-Francis E. *Global Health Disparities. Closing the gap through good governance*. Sudbury, MA: Jones and Bartlett Learning; 2011.

Lalonde M. *A New Perspective on the Health of Canadians*. Ottawa: National Health and Welfare; 1974.

Raziz DV. The risk of a sixth mass extinction of life and the role of medicine. *J R Soc Med*. 2010; **103**: 473–4.

Roberts I. Fat chance for Cancun. *J R Soc Med*. 2011; **104**: 43–4.

Sachs J. *The End of Poverty*. London: Penguin Books; 2005.

Setel PW, Macfarlane SB, Szreter S, *et al*, on behalf of the Monitoring of Vital Events (MoVE) Writing Group. A scandal of invisibility: making everyone count by counting everyone. *Lancet*. 2007; **370**: 1726–35.

Stuckler D, Basu S, Suhrcke M, *et al*. The public health effect of economic crises and alternative policy responses in Europe: an empirical evaluation. *Lancet*. 2009; **374**: 315–23.

Suhrcke M, McKee M, Sauto Arce R, *et al*. *The Contribution of Health to the Economy in the European Union*. Brussels: European Commission; 2005.

Wilkinson R, Pickett K. *The Spirit Level: why equality is better for everyone*. London: Penguin Books; 2010.

Wolinsky SM. Preface. In: Garrett L. *Betrayal of Trust: the collapse of global public health*. New York: Hyperion; 2000. p.xiii.

World Health Organization. *Alma-Ata. Primary Health Care* (Health for All Series No. 1). Geneva: World Health Organization; 1978.

World Health Organization/World Bank. *World Report on Disability*. Geneva: World Health Organization; 2011.

CHAPTER 2

Taking a closer look: the changing global burden of disease

COMBINING MORTALITY AND MORBIDITY: THE GLOBAL BURDEN OF DISEASE

The burden of disease on the population is the impact of that disease, in a defined geographical area, measured by financial cost, mortality, morbidity or other indicators. Simply describing a population exclusively in terms of its mortality feels intuitively unsatisfactory. First, we all die some time so death in itself is not necessarily 'unhealthy'. What we really need is a measure of premature death, such as the number of years of life lost (YLL), preferably broken down into specific causes. Second, death is only the tip of the pyramid of population ill health and has to be complemented by morbidity and quality of life data. These are scarce and, where they do exist, are seldom easily related either to a time scale, i.e. whether the illness is short-lived (acute) or long-standing (disability), or to mortality. Ideally, we need an indicator of population health that encompasses mortality (from all causes and cause specific), acute morbidity and disability, all in relation to age and preferably to gender and other variables as well. Does such an indicator exist? There have been several attempts to create one.

The construction of a summary indicator of population health that takes account of both mortality and morbidity (including disability) has been the holy grail of epidemiologists for decades. Several early attempts were discarded either because they were too expensive (being dependent on detailed questionnaire-based population surveys) or because they proved difficult to disaggregate into causal categories, severity and age groups, or for other technical reasons. One promising indicator was the Health-Adjusted Life Expectancy (HALE) that seeks to summarise the expected number of years to be lived in what might be termed the equivalent of good health. The HALE is calculated by subtracting from the overall life expectancy the number of years of ill health, weighted for severity.

Two further indicators jostled for pre-eminence in the world of burden-of-disease methodology. These were quality-adjusted life-years (QALYs) and disability-adjusted life-years (DALYs); both combine the burden due to death and morbidity into one index. They allow for comparisons of the disease burden due to various risk factors or diseases and also make it possible to predict the possible impact of health interventions. Of these, the DALY has become increasingly popular, with the encouragement of the World Health Organization (WHO) and the World Bank. It combines both mortality and morbidity and takes account of both the years of life lost prematurely (YLL) and those years of life lived but blighted by disability (YLD). It is an extension of potential years of life lost (derived by subtracting age of death from life expectancy). It takes account of quality of life by applying an illness and disability weighting to the YLL through premature death, using the 'healthiest' possible population (such as Japan) as the benchmark. It is calculated, as shown in this equation, by adding the YLL to the years of life lived (or healthy years of life lost) with disability (YLD):

DALY = YLL + YLD

Years of life lost is an aggregate of the ages of deaths of victims subtracted from the average life expectancy of that population; YLD is calculated by applying a disability weighting to the aggregated years lived by victims from the diagnosis of the disease to death. The disability weightings are derived either from empirical research or from the judgement of an expert panel. One DALY may be regarded as the equivalent of one healthy year of life lost. The result is that the DALY tends to give greater weight to deaths at younger ages though it measures much more than premature death. An alternative measure, disability-free life expectancy (DFLE), gives an indication of the quality of any extra years of life. It is said to be more objective than the DALY as it doesn't rely on a disability weighting based on expert opinion. Unfortunately, DFLE has a limited utility due to the need for repeated disability surveys over time in countries that are being compared (Beaglehole and Bonita 1997).

The DALY can be viewed as a composite measure that adds together the losses of healthy years of life attributable to illness, disability and death. It also 'discounts' future losses, regarding them as worth less than losses occurring today. This novel methodology was applied to all regions and most countries of the world in the ground-breaking WHO-sponsored Global Burden of Disease (GBD) study (Murray and Lopez 1996). The GBD study documented, for the first time, international comparisons of over 100 diseases and injuries, plus 10 major risk factors, using a common metric that simultaneously accounted for both premature mortality and morbidity (prevalence, duration and severity of non-fatal disease). The impact of this ambitious, if controversial, analysis on global public health was profound (Mathers 2007). It demonstrated with much more clarity than hitherto the striking variations in health between countries and regions. It also highlighted the huge burden of mental illness and injuries, both of which are responsible for a relatively small proportion of deaths alongside a relatively large toll of disability. These two groups of disorders had been previously underestimated when mortality rates alone were analysed.

On publication of these results, countries and regions were able to benchmark, in some detail, their relative successes and failures, as reflected in these population health indicators, against each other. That was a major advance for the global public health community. Yet reservations about the GBD approach were numerous and sometimes stridently expressed. Critics focused on three main aspects: its methodology, its application and its philosophical basis (Mathers 2007). Methodological concerns related to the construction and underlying assumptions of DALYs, including the extrapolation of an individual health status measure to whole populations, the specific disability and age weighting methods, the paucity of evidence about their validity and reliability, their relatively narrow focus on individual health rather than the wider impact of the disorder on families and communities, and the incompleteness of available data around the world. GBD estimates of mental illness, for example, have been criticised for the poor quality of the underlying data (Brhlikova *et al* 2011).

Other writers worried about the use (or misuse) of the GBD approach for policy making, arguing, for example, that priorities should reflect the cost-effectiveness of interventions rather than the epidemiological magnitude of diseases (Mooney *et al* 1997) though there is no obvious reason why these two dimensions should not be reconciled. Finally, there is ongoing controversy around the meaning and appropriateness of the disability component. Some lobby groups strongly object to the inclusion of disability at all in the GBD equation, arguing that this signifies a return to an era of allegedly 'medical model' stigmatisation of people with disabilities who are, it is claimed, just as likely to be 'healthy' as their able-bodied counterparts.

Bearing in mind the various reservations, what do these analyses tell us about the current state of health of the world's population in relation to the past?

Global Burden of Disease study findings

Deaths

In 2004, an estimated 58.8 million deaths occurred worldwide (Mathers *et al* 2008). Of these, just over half (53%) were in males. The median age of death was (approximately) 60 years and the global average was 66. The highest age-adjusted death rates were reported from the poorest regions (Figure 2.1; *see* colour plate section between pages 46 and 47). This is reflected in life expectancy that ranged from almost 80 years in high-income countries to below 50 years in Africa, a 60% difference. Life expectancy increased in the preceding decade or so in most regions of the world with the exception of Africa and Eastern Europe.

Deaths by cause and gender

The GBD study groups the data into three causal categories: communicable, reproductive or nutritional disorders (Group 1); non-communicable, mostly chronic disease (Group 2); and injuries, whether unintentional or intentional (Group 3). Although Group 1 conditions occur mainly in poorer countries, most (60%) deaths in 2004 were due to Group 2 conditions, 30% were due to Group 1 conditions, and 10% were due to Group 3 conditions. Cardiovascular diseases (mainly ischaemic heart and cerebrovascular) were the leading cause of death, particularly among women, followed by infections (especially respiratory and diarrhoeal), cancer (notably of the lung, breast and digestive tract) and respiratory diseases. Road casualties were the main cause of injury deaths. The leading causes of death in high-income countries were cardiovascular disease, cancer and chronic obstructive lung disease. In low-income countries, the leading causes of death were infections, neonatal causes and HIV/AIDS. The gender ratio was roughly equal for most causes, with the notable exception of injuries, in which males predominated, though it should be noted that the gender pattern of deaths varies by age (see next section).

An updated report on the causes of death (World Health Organization 2011) observed that 36 million, or almost two-thirds, of the 57 million deaths that occurred globally in 2008 were in the non-communicable (Group 2) category. These were mainly cardiovascular diseases, cancers, diabetes and chronic lung diseases. In turn, these deaths were attributable to four main risk factors associated with economic transition, urbanisation and the 21st-century lifestyle: tobacco use, unhealthy diet, insufficient physical activity and harmful use of alcohol.

Deaths by age

In 2004, almost a fifth of all deaths were in children under the age of five. Nearly three-quarters of the 10.4 million deaths in this age group were due to six causes: acute respiratory infections, mainly pneumonia (17%), diarrhoeal diseases (17%), prematurity and low birthweight (11%), neonatal infections (9%), birth asphyxia and trauma (8%), and malaria (7%). The age distribution of deaths varied starkly between regions. There was a 25-fold variation in under-five child mortality between regions, largely due to the varying levels of communicable diseases, poverty and malnutrition. In high-income countries, only 1% of deaths were children under 15 while 84% were people aged 60 and over. In low-income regions, the pattern is reversed: 46% of all deaths were children under 15 whereas only 20% were people aged 60 and over. Africa was particularly affected by child deaths: more than 90% of under-five deaths in the world that are attributable to malaria occurred there, and the figure is similar for HIV/AIDS deaths. If all countries had the child mortality rates of Japan (the lowest in the world), only 1 million child deaths rather than 10 million would occur each year.

Adult (15–59 years) mortality was highest in Africa (due mainly to Group 1 causes), followed by Europe (due mainly to Group 2 causes). In all regions, adult mortality rates were higher in males than in females. Male adult mortality was notably high in Eastern Europe, while in the African region women had a higher mortality than men due to Group 2 causes. Injuries and cardiovascular diseases were the leading causes of death in European men. And injuries were the main causes of death in adult men in Latin America, the Caribbean and Eastern Mediterranean regions. Using the YLL indicator, the pattern shifts somewhat. Group 2 (non-communicable) diseases become less important, while the relative importance of Africa and South-East Asia becomes greater because of the younger age at death in these regions.

Global burden of morbidity and disability

By their nature, estimates of morbidity and disability are much less certain than those of mortality. In 2004, diarrhoea was believed to be the most common cause of episodes of illness (incidence) in the world followed by lower respiratory infections. The most prevalent morbid condition was thought to be iron deficiency anaemia (1.1 billion) followed by hearing loss (636 million) and migraine (324 million). Poor vision or blindness (315 million), asthma (235 million) and diabetes mellitus (221 million) were not far behind.

Using GBD definitions based on 'loss of health' or functioning capacity, 15% of the world's population were estimated to suffer from moderate or severe disability, ranging from 5% in children to 46% in the over-60s. In all age groups, the prevalence of disability was higher in poorer than affluent countries. Females had a slightly higher rate of severe disability. Visual and hearing disorders, followed by mental disorders and injuries, were estimated to be the leading causes of moderate and severe disability. Neuropsychiatric disorders (especially depression) and sensory disorders dominated the impact of disability as measured by YLD and accounted for a third of YLD among adults. The burden of depression was 50% higher for females than males. The pattern was similar for other psychiatric disorders including dementia. By contrast, the burden for alcohol and drug disorders was nearly seven times higher for males than for females.

In reviewing the GBD study, Mathers (2007) observed that the 'epidemiological transition' (see below) in poorer countries resulted in a 20% reduction in the 1990s in the *per capita* disease burden due to communicable, maternal and perinatal, and nutritional disorders. This impressive figure would have been greater still (around 30%) had it not been for the impact of the

HIV/AIDS epidemic, because of its direct effects on mortality and its indirect effects via traditional infections such as tuberculosis (TB) and malaria that disproportionately affect people with immune systems weakened by HIV/AIDS. Mathers described the 'triple burden' facing poorer regions in the form of the old infectious diseases plus the emerging epidemics of chronic non-communicable diseases (including mental illness and injuries) plus the new health threats associated with globalisation and climate change. These phenomena are observable not only in the shifting pattern of mortality rates but also in a 'risk factor transition' whereby 'affluent' factors such as smoking, alcohol and overweight are increasingly impacting on poorer countries (see below).

Global burden of disability-adjusted life-years
Disability-adjusted life-years (the loss of equivalent years of full health) permit a comparison of the burden of disease across conditions that cause varying levels of mortality and disability. Globally, 60% of DALYs in 2004 were due to premature mortality and 40% were due to non-fatal health outcomes. DALYs affected Africa and South-East Asia disproportionately; in Africa DALYs were at least double those in any other region, with YLL rates seven times higher than in high-income countries. Group 1 (infectious) disorders accounted for the greatest inter-regional variation, with poorer regions especially affected, yet Group 2 (non-communicable) diseases by now accounted for almost half the burden of disease in poorer countries. This is probably due to population ageing and changes in the prevalence of risk factors in many regions. Non-communicable diseases dominated the burden in high-income countries due mainly to their older populations. European low- and middle-income countries had the highest proportion (16%) of burden due to injuries. Globally, men aged 15–44 appeared at particularly high risk from injuries. Poisoning was a notable cause of injury death in poorer European countries while death rates through fires were higher for women in South-East Asia than for men or women in other regions. Children bore more than half of the disease burden in poorer countries.

The top 10 causes of the burden of disease (DALYs) in 2004 were:
1   lower respiratory infection
2   diarrhoeal diseases
3   unipolar depressive disorders
4   ischaemic heart disease
5   HIV/AIDS
6   cerebrovascular disease
7   prematurity and low birthweight
8   birth asphyxia and trauma
9   road traffic accidents
10 neonatal infections.

Depression was ranked third worldwide and eighth in low-income countries. It was the leading cause among young adult women (15–44 years). Cigarette smoking and alcohol are major contributors to several of these disorders.

Global health risks

As mentioned earlier, the GBD study has also attempted to quantify the contribution of underlying risk factors to global mortality and disability (World Health Organization 2009). The findings varied somewhat according to the study period and the outcome measures used. The leading global health risks for mortality in 2004 were high blood pressure (responsible for 13% of deaths globally), tobacco use (9%), high blood glucose (6%), physical inactivity (6%), and overweight and obesity (5%). The leading risks for disease burden as measured by DALYs were underweight (6% of global DALYs), unsafe sex (5%), alcohol use (5%), and unsafe water, sanitation and hygiene. These findings may be summarised as follows: five leading risk factors (childhood underweight, unsafe sex, alcohol use, unsafe water and sanitation, and high blood pressure) were responsible for a quarter of all deaths and a fifth of all DALYs. These estimates were derived from calculations of the population-attributable fraction – the proportional reduction in population disease or mortality that would occur if exposure to that risk factor was reduced to an alternative ideal exposure level.

As a country develops economically and its population ages, it undergoes the 'risk transition' (in parallel with the epidemiological transition) whereby the pattern of risk factors shifts from those associated with poverty (e.g. childhood underweight, poor sanitation) to those associated with affluence (e.g. tobacco, obesity). Keeping track of the risk transition is important as it enables epidemiologists to predict with greater certainty what the future burden of disease in a particular country or region is likely to be. It also helps policy makers to undertake anticipatory planning of public health interventions designed to control the risk factors, prevent the associated diseases and disorders, and provide appropriate healthcare for patients.

TIME TRENDS IN THE GLOBAL BURDEN OF DISEASE STUDY

One way of monitoring time trends in global health is to compare successive analyses of the GBD study. The 1990 estimates were revised in later analyses for 2001 (Lopez *et al* 2006) and 2004 (Mathers *et al* 2008, Mathers and Bonita 2009). The three are not strictly comparable due to methodological refinements, especially in the quantification of risk factors and their contribution to mortality. Nevertheless, some interesting time trends in the overall patterns are perceptible and are probably real rather than artefactual.

A major geographical shift in the GBD occurred between the first two GBD analyses. In Eastern Europe/Central Asia, the *per capita* disease burden (with associated reductions in life expectancy) increased by nearly 40% between 1990 and 2001, pushing this region into third place in the poor health league after South Asia and sub-Saharan Africa. This seems to reflect rising rates of alcohol abuse, suicide and violence in countries that have been experiencing major social, political and economic upheaval.

Repeated GBD analyses have shown that the precise composition and ranking of conditions vary over time. Examples of this reordering are unipolar depression and road traffic injuries, both of which rose up the rankings between 1990 and 2004. More important, perhaps, than the ranking of specific disorders is the general pattern: we see a mix of communicable and chronic diseases (including mental illness), each contributing around half of total DALYs. The former tend to dominate the picture in low- and middle-income countries while the latter are more noteworthy in high-income countries. Road traffic injuries impose a major burden across the globe and are expected to rise up the rankings in the future.

Global under-five years mortality is decreasing and is expected to have declined by 27% from 1990 to 2015. Though this falls short of the Millennium Development Goal 4 target of 67%, it is nevertheless a major achievement. Renewed efforts will be needed to address diarrhoeal diseases, pneumonia, malaria and neonatal deaths. In adults, a particular cause for concern is cancer. In 2004, out of 7.4 million deaths due to cancer, there were around 1.32 million deaths (18% of the total) from lung cancer, a 40% increase since 1990 reflecting rising smoking rates in poorer countries. Three-quarters of these occurred in men. Stomach cancer, previously the leading malignant cause of death, declined globally in all regions. In women, breast cancer was the most common malignancy followed by respiratory tract and stomach cancer.

The GBD analyses epitomise the highly sophisticated way in which modern epidemiologists describe patterns of health and disease across the world. Some of these patterns relate to geography, age, gender, social class or time. Time trends are particularly fascinating and important because they tell us something about our past successes and failures, help us make predictions about the future and inform decision making in the present. But are we any closer to understanding the underlying reasons for these patterns? Epidemiologists have struggled hard to answer this question and have offered some tentative if partial explanations. Epidemiology is especially well suited to making temporal observations. To make more sense of the changing nature of global health over time, as well as our attempts to respond to it effectively, it is helpful to take account of some epidemiological concepts that may be described as the three transitions: the demographic transition, the epidemiological transition and the sustainability transition.

The demographic transition

For at least the past two centuries, demographers have predicted an exponential rise in the world's population to the point where the sustainability of human life becomes questionable. The first alarm bells were set ringing in the late 18th century by Thomas Malthus (1798), who predicted that population growth would generate severe poverty and would thus always be limited by famine, pestilence and other catastrophes. Malthusian ideas were highly influential over the succeeding century and a half. His theme was embellished and dramatised in the 20th century by Ehrlich (1968) who warned of the inevitability of hundreds of millions of deaths through famine in the 1970s due to overpopulation if evasive action, including mandatory birth control if necessary, was not taken urgently.

We now have the luxury of hindsight with which to test these doom-laden prognoses. What actually happened? The world's population has certainly increased steeply since Malthus's time. But Armageddon didn't sweep away the human race though there have been periodic setbacks in the form of world wars, natural disasters, famine and disease. Although many poorer countries have struggled to meet the needs of their rapidly increasing populations, we can take some comfort from the fact that the direst consequences of demographic growth that Malthus, Ehrlich and their followers predicted simply failed to materialise. This was almost certainly due to the remarkable development of agricultural technology combined with environmental, social and public health (including healthcare) advances. That doesn't mean that the dangers of overpopulation have evaporated. What happened in the past may be a poor guide to what will happen in the future.

The changing demographic composition of the population is as (and in some circumstances more) important than its absolute size. The dynamic and predictable nature of this changing structure, along with its social, political and health implications, has to be taken into account by public health planners. The American demographer Warren Thompson summarised the phenomenon in two words: *demographic transition* (DT). In essence, the DT model describes the evolution of countries over many decades in terms of some key demographic features. Prior to the DT, countries typically have high birth and death rates, resulting in fairly slow population growth (if any). As they move through the DT, countries exhibit declining death rates followed (after a few years) by declining birth rates as people respond to a lower risk of infant and child death by reducing family size. The net initial result is an increase in population, starting with a higher proportion of children and young people, as is happening today in many poor regions. As fertility declines and the population ages, the proportion of older people increases, a phenomenon familiar today to most affluent and many middle-income countries. These demographic changes are the outcome of a complex and interacting series of influences that exert their

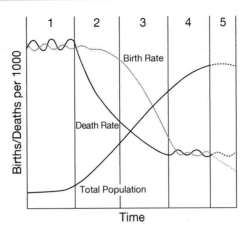

Figure 2.2 The demographic transition. Source: Wikipedia: http://en.wikipedia.org/wiki/ Demographic_transition. Copyright Wikimedia Commons: http://creativecommons.org/ licenses/by-sa/3.0/

effects as countries move from an agrarian or at least preindustrial economy to an industrialised one. And the impact of these changes on societies is far-reaching, economically, industrially, socially and culturally.

There are several stages to the DT (Figure 2.2).

➤ In *stage 1*, birth and death rates are both high and this produces a steady state with a stable population.

➤ In *stage 2*, death rates fall due to improving nutrition, sanitation and education. Because birth rates remain high, the total population expands.

➤ In *stage 3*, birth rates fall due to contraception, urbanisation and female employment. At this point the population starts to fall.

➤ In *stage 4*, a combination of low birth and death rates leads again to a stable population for a substantial period of time.

➤ In *stage 5*, low fertility leads to population shrinkage and an increasing economic burden placed by dependent age groups (especially older people) on the working population.

Most developing countries are working their way through the first two stages while industrialised countries have reached the latter two. The DT has a variable time scale and it seems to be accelerating. Some previously extremely poor countries and regions (such as Asia) have progressed extremely rapidly through nearly all the stages while others (such as sub-Saharan Africa) have stalled at stages 1, 2 or 3.

The DT may be regarded as both a blessing and a curse. The first three stages are clearly liberating for a population while the fourth produces a whole new set of problems. In high- and middle-income countries, the demographic threat arises less from numerical trends than shifting age distributions. The demographic pyramid becomes top heavy, with a relatively large older segment of the population, with its accompanying health and social dependencies, exerting an ever-increasing burden on their younger working counterparts. To put it another way, the net income-generating (through tax contributions) sector of the population risks being overwhelmed by the net income-consuming (through public service usage) one. Japan, for example, is thought to be the most rapidly ageing country in the world, suffering from a combination of declining population, a rising proportion of older people and overburdened public services. To some extent, sustained economic growth may compensate for this imbalance but that cannot be relied upon as the most recent (2008–9) of the periodic global economic recessions has demonstrated.

Echoes of Malthus and Ehrlich nevertheless still resonate in the 21st century though demographic concerns have taken on a novel form. The imminent occurrence of catastrophe is again being predicted, not so much on the basis of fears of a population explosion brought about by the demographic 'time bomb' but from concerns about the long-term sustainability of even the current world population. Environmentalists warn that the earth simply cannot support the current population, let alone an ever-expanding one, without inflicting lethal damage to the atmosphere and ecosystem to the point where life itself is placed in jeopardy. A closely linked concern is that relating to climate change and its consequences for agriculture, the food supply and the transport infrastructure. Sharply rising food prices, in particular, will impact most strongly on precisely those families and communities that are already struggling to stave off malnutrition. The language may be less cataclysmic but the intense anxiety remains.

In summary: the past 200 years have brought both good and bad demographic news. Although Malthusian calamities have been avoided, the world population is still increasing fast, its size and ageing structure are unsustainable, and these factors collectively pose a very real threat to human quality of life as well as survival. Not all regions of the world are equally affected: population growth has been happening much faster in poorer countries due to lack of education, poor contraceptive services, cultural attitudes that favour large families, and high infant mortality rates that reinforce the tendency to high fertility. There are exceptions, China being the most notable due to its controversial one-child policy, but the pattern of disproportionate population growth in those countries least able to afford it is nevertheless a real one. By contrast, population contraction, a characteristic of the latter stages of the demographic transition in wealthier countries, carries its own risks to human health and welfare and is compounded by the economic stresses caused by a top-heavy demographic pyramid.

The epidemiological transition

The epidemiological transition (ET), sometimes called the health transition, runs in parallel with the DT, characterised by falling birth and death rates, and is an elaboration of the DT in that it focuses on the causes of death in a population that contribute to demographic change (Omran 1971). The ET simply means the change in the pattern of disease that occurs when a population moves from a relatively poor agrarian-based economy to a relatively rich industrialised one. In the former scenario, malnutrition and infections dominate the picture of mortality and morbidity while in the latter, chronic diseases and trauma come to the fore. People living in countries that have undergone the ET generally have a higher standard of living, better health and a longer life expectancy than those living in countries that have not. The ET, like the DT, is not an event but a process that unfolds over many decades, though the time scale varies greatly from country to country. The ET is caused, in part, by the changing pattern of risks to which a population undergoing economic development is exposed – the so-called 'risk transition' (see above).

In theory, therefore, the ET, like the DT, is a phenomenon to be welcomed around the world as it should herald better health and wellbeing for all. Sadly, as in the case of the DT, the reality is usually rather different. Many developing countries that are currently undergoing the ET seem to have stuttered to a halt in mid-process with the result that they are experiencing the worst of both worlds – high levels of malnutrition and infection combined with high levels of chronic disease and trauma. The emergence of many of the 'Western' diseases in low-income countries, such as lung cancer, coronary heart disease and stroke, is attributable both to lifestyle changes consequent upon economic development and to the deliberate and cynical marketing of tobacco, alcohol and other potentially damaging products to large new markets. Others, such as road traffic casualties and interpersonal violence, reflect increasing motorisation and urbanisation, phenomena that are also closely correlated with economic development and a shift towards patterns of living and environmental conditions that are familiar to residents of affluent countries.

Simultaneously, a number of relatively affluent post-ET populations (such as the countries of the former Soviet Union) seem to have slipped backwards into an era of new nutritional and infectious threats (notably obesity, HIV, tuberculosis and multiply resistant microbial infections) while being unable either to solve their continuing epidemics of chronic disease, trauma and mental illness, or to reduce the ubiquitous social inequalities in health in their populations. And as mortality rates decline, it seems theoretically plausible that morbidity and disability rates will increase as people survive longer while suffering from diseases of ageing – so-called *morbidity expansion* (Fries 1980). Against this, improvements in population health might, equally plausibly, be expected to result in longer, healthier lives – so-called *morbidity compression*

(Fries 2003). Which of these two contradictory phenomena will ultimately predominate remains unclear although it is likely that the former will pose the greater short-term challenge.

The epidemiological transition in a high-income country: the case of the United Kingdom

The United Kingdom is one of the most affluent countries in the world and is widely envied for its mature liberal democracy, its mixed economy and highly developed health, welfare and educational systems. Despite impressive improvements in health indicators such as infant mortality and life expectancy, it continues to mount an apparently unproductive struggle against several seemingly intractable health problems. Paramount among these is the health gap between rich and poor. Successive British governments since the Second World War have failed to reduce the persistent and sometimes widening social inequalities in health despite increasingly determined attempts to do so. In that sense, the UK is typical of many high-income countries. Its recent epidemiological experience is instructive.

Over the last two centuries, enormous social and cultural changes have transformed the country, usually as a result of major international events to which Britain, as an agricultural island trading nation, was especially vulnerable. Following the Industrial Revolution in the 19th century, its burgeoning urban population placed intolerable strains on the national economy that ultimately led to periods of prolonged unemployment, poverty and wide social inequalities. These negative trends were exacerbated by a residual yet extremely brittle social class structure that limited educational opportunities for children of disadvantaged backgrounds, and a relentless postindustrial economic decline in areas that had once been exclusively dependent on heavy engineering, coal mining and other rapidly shrinking sources of employment. Added to those difficulties must be counted the massive politico-economic setback resulting from the loss of Empire in the 20th century and the corrosive effects of prolonged periods of violent conflict, the most notable being the two World Wars.

Against this bleak picture must be set several opposing, health-promoting trends. Among these were major enlightened societal initiatives including the introduction of the welfare state and the NHS in the first half of the 20th century. These, combined with steadily rising living standards, resulted in a sustained era of political stability as the nation adjusted to peaceful co-existence with its immediate neighbours and came to terms with its postcolonial status. Despite intermittent periods of economic austerity, the country generally prospered and invested heavily in its public services, including the NHS, housing and education. The overall result of these multiple and interacting social, political and healthcare factors was a major shift in the pattern of health that accords with the descriptor 'epidemiological transition'.

The UK seems to have undergone the ET around the Second World War though it is difficult to pinpoint a precise date on what was, as indicated earlier, a long-term process rather than a one-off event. The ET should have been good news for the UK, especially as declining mortality rates led to increased life expectancy. In general terms, it undoubtedly was. Yet the state of UK population health continues to this day to cause serious concern to professionals, the public and governments. That is attributable to two key phenomena: the emergence of new epidemics of both infectious and chronic diseases (notably antibiotic-resistant infections and obesity), and widening social inequalities in health.

One of the central difficulties in interpreting the ET and secular (long-term time) health trends in general is that we are uncertain what causes them. The dramatic improvements in life expectancy and the reduction in infant mortality in Western Europe between the early 18th and mid-20th centuries were almost entirely a reflection of the decline of infectious diseases such as small-pox, measles, typhoid, cholera and tuberculosis (McKeown 1976). That begs the question: what caused that decline? Was it due to better sanitation, cleaner water, more spacious housing? Was it the introduction of vaccines for small-pox, poliomyelitis (polio) and tuberculosis or did these specific preventive weapons arrive too late, as McKeown asserted, to make a major contribution? Did the organisms themselves mutate into less lethal forms? Was the immune status of the population improving through better nutrition? Was medical care becoming more rational and effective? Was it a combination of all of these factors? (Chapter 5 discusses these questions further.)

We can garner some evidence that might explain the historical record of affluent countries from the recent experience of poorer countries. McMichael and Beaglehole (2009) believe that the decline in mortality in the latter is best explained by improvements in three areas: rising household incomes leading to better material conditions and nutrition; educational development, especially schooling for girls that enhances gender equality, leading to improved maternal and child health; and the diffusion of scientific, technological and practical knowledge, producing more effective and efficient healthcare and preventive interventions.

Many low-income countries are currently undergoing the ET while others have scarcely embarked on the journey. Garrett (2000) suggests that the ones left behind constitute a majority and judges their governments' records harshly.

> For most of the world's population in 2000, the public health essentials mapped out in New York before World War 1 have never existed: progress, in the form of safe water, food, housing, sewage, and hospitals, has never come. An essential trust, between government and its people, in pursuit of health for all has never been established. In other parts of the world – notably the former Soviet Union – the trust was long ago betrayed.

The ET, like the DT, is more than a statistical model of past events. It clarifies historical trends in a way that has major implications for current and future public health policy. A key challenge for rich countries is to work out how to steer poor countries through these transitions more quickly and in a manner that is sustainable, in terms of both affordability and environmental impact.

The sustainability transition

At the start of the third millennium, a new concept began to evolve that took account of the demographic and epidemiological transitions but looked forward to an era of international action encapsulated in the phrase *sustainability transition* (ST). McMichael *et al* (2000) eloquently summarised the challenge.

Meanwhile, a further set of large-scale environmental problems has emerged and moved towards centre-stage. They add up to the conviction that we are living beyond the Earth's means, and that the continued increase in human numbers and economic activity poses a serious problem for the world as a whole. In September 1999 the United Nations Environment Programme (UNEP) issued its global environment outlook 2000, whose final chapter begins as follows.

> The beginning of a new millennium finds the planet Earth poised between two conflicting trends. A wasteful and invasive consumer society, coupled with continued population growth, is threatening to destroy the resources on which human life is based. At the same time, society is locked in a struggle against time to reverse these trends and introduce sustainable practices that will ensure the welfare of future generations. (United Nations Environment Programme 1999)

It goes almost without saying that global health is dependent on the preservation of the earth's vital resources. Human disruption to the environment, according to McMichael and colleagues, arises from three interdependent sources: population size, levels of material consumption and production, and technology. All three require careful planning, managing and monitoring. Globalisation, whether economic, technological or cultural, has produced undoubted benefits but we are moving into an era in which the growing human population is exerting unbearable strain on the natural environment. Potentially damaging global environmental changes (GECs) include disturbances in atmospheric gas composition, soil degradation, food and water shortages, deforestation, desertification, reduced biodiversity and chemical pollution. All GECs have major negative implications for public health.

The major threat to the environment today is probably climate change and associated phenomena caused by the massive rise in carbon dioxide emissions in the 20th century (*see* Chapter 15). Apart from a small minority of sceptics, most informed scientific opinion accepts that statement. By the end of the

21st century, the Intergovernmental Panel on Climate Change (2007) predicts a rise in global temperature of up to 6°C (though somewhere in the range between 2°C and 4°C may be more likely). The increased risks to health that this will cause include more frequent severe weather events, increasing incidence of vector-borne infections (such as malaria, dengue fever and leishmaniasis), food-borne and water-borne diseases, skin cancer and eye disease due to depletion of stratospheric ozone, declining agricultural yields, salination of coastal regions and freshwater supplies due to sea-level rise, and a multiplicity of other effects. All parts of the world and all communities are likely to be affected albeit to varying degrees. This process needs to be reversed urgently to avoid destroying the ecosystems on which humanity depends. The ST is not, then, so much a historical phenomenon as a contemporary imperative. Unlike the two previous transitions, the ST will not happen unless we ensure that it does by promoting ecologically sustainable social and ecological development (*see* Chapters 10 and 15).

TIME TRENDS IN GLOBAL HEALTH: FOR BETTER OR FOR WORSE?

So, taking account of all these time trends, where are we now? The answer has to be guarded. The future is simply too hard to predict with any degree of certainty. Nevertheless, it would be wise to take seriously the possibility, at the very least, that humanity faces potential disaster, whether mediated by population growth, the demographic transition, environmental damage or climate change (or all of these). Demographers continue to warn of the dangers of overpopulation and ageing in some regions, interacting with environmental degradation and climate change, even if their strictures are becoming increasingly nuanced. The strong scientific consensus around the fact of climate change, and its potential consequences, is not matched by one relating either to its causes or solutions. Nevertheless, the vast majority of countries now recognise the need to reduce carbon and greenhouse gas emissions even if actions fall short of stated aspirations. International mechanisms for achieving more effective interventions seem to be slowly bearing fruit. Equally, technology may again rescue the earth from population growth and its consequences. Several of these issues are discussed in greater depth later in this book.

This complex state of affairs may be summed up as follows: huge progress has been made, for reasons that are incompletely understood, but the picture is variable, with some large regions showing signs of deteriorating health. Moreover, those achievements that have been observed may turn out to have been fragile and temporary as a result of newly arising threats from shifting demographic patterns, epidemiological setbacks in the control of both communicable and chronic diseases, and global environmental disruption. Despite the suppression of previously lethal diseases and the prolongation of life expectancy in many countries, numerous seemingly intractable health problems remain – and may be worsening – in both developed and developing countries. The temporal improvement in global population health has been unequivocal and should not be underestimated but we should also bear in mind that some of it may be transient, reversible or, in a worst-case scenario, entirely illusory.

SOME SPECIFIC DISEASE CHALLENGES
Infectious disease
The GBD estimates demonstrate the continuing importance of infection as a cause of death and disability worldwide. It remains a major cause of death in poor countries and is the most important contributor to burden of disease in sub-Saharan Africa. Skolnik (2008) has drawn attention to the large numbers of people killed annually by a handful of diseases:
➤ HIV/AIDS 3 million
➤ diarrhoea 1.8 million
➤ tuberculosis 1.6 million
➤ malaria 1.2 million.

Three features of communicable diseases are especially noteworthy: they affect children in huge numbers, are associated with poverty and are often preventable. Seven out of 10 deaths in children under five occur in low-income countries (Mathers and Bonita 2009). These deaths are attributable to just five preventable diseases: respiratory infections, diarrhoea, malaria, measles and malnutrition. Only the last is non-infectious but it contributes enormously, in synergy with poverty, to increased susceptibility to infection. Measles, for example, is a more serious disease in malnourished children, especially those who are deficient in vitamin A. The death rate from measles is under 3 per 1000 cases in high-income countries while in poorer regions it is 10 or even 100 times higher. Other infections associated with poverty include skin and eye infections and hepatitis. Over 2 billion people worldwide are infected with the hepatitis B virus, which causes over a million deaths a year. Children may be victims of mother-to-baby hepatitis transmission and become chronic (usually undiagnosed) carriers, leading to an elevated risk later in life of liver cirrhosis or cancer.

Infections are often thought of as being short-lived but they can have serious long-term consequences even if the disease itself has a brief course. Apart from the toll of suffering they cause to the victims and their families as a result of complications such as brain damage and other forms of disability, they hinder the physical and mental development of children, impair their educational progress and undermine their future economic prospects. Adult sufferers of recurrent or chronic infections are often incapable of sustained employment and place a strain on family, community and national resources. The tragedy of this situation is that so many of these diseases can be prevented or cured. And indeed, much of the world has succeeded in substantially reducing the toll of death and disability from infections. Unfortunately, progress in controlling communicable diseases, both in children and the general population, in many countries has been halted and even reversed by a resurgence of old diseases, notably malaria and tuberculosis (Figure 2.3; *see* colour plate section between pages 46 and 47), and by the emergence of some new ones, particularly the human immunodeficiency virus. Of the roughly 34 million people with HIV/AIDS, 95% live in low- and middle-income countries, the majority in sub-Saharan Africa. And HIV infection greatly increases susceptibility to other infections such as tuberculosis. That is why these 'big three' communicable diseases have become the target of concerted international efforts to reduce their incidence, prevalence and impact.

Chronic disease

All three of the major killers – cancer, cardiovascular disorders and respiratory disease – in adult life are caused, at least in part, by cigarette smoking. Although its prevalence has declined in most affluent countries, it continues to rise in poorer ones. There are about 6 million tobacco-related deaths each year (about half of which occur in low-income countries), a figure that is expected to rise to 8.4 million by 2030 (Mathers and Loncar 2006). Over a billion people smoke worldwide, most of whom are men, and there is an inverse correlation between socioeconomic status and the extent of smoking. Like alcohol misuse, smoking is an addiction, with origins in childhood and adolescence, which casts a long shadow in terms of ill health across the entire life cycle.

Apart from tobacco, demographic change is generating ever greater burdens of ill health around the world. The ageing of the population is associated with inevitable rises in the incidence and prevalence of chronic diseases such as heart disease, stroke, cancers, diabetes, chronic respiratory disease, arthritis, sensory deficits and dementia. These disorders are widely considered to afflict affluent populations particularly but they are also increasingly making their presence felt in poor countries as they move through the epidemiological transition. Because of the demographic drift towards an older population across the globe, non-communicable diseases are steadily supplanting infections as the world's leading cause of death and are now thought to account for two-thirds of deaths globally, with 80% occurring in low- and middle-income countries. By 2030, it is predicted that three-quarters of all deaths will be due to this group of conditions. The good news is that chronic disease mortality has been declining for several decades in affluent countries, probably due to the improved control of risk factors such as smoking, high blood pressure and high blood cholesterol combined with more effective treatments, including surgery. That trend may not continue in the future as all countries try to cope with rapidly rising rates of overweight and obesity.

Obesity

Once considered a disease of affluence, caused by a combination of a sedentary lifestyle and overconsumption of high-energy food, obesity is now a global pandemic. An INSERM survey (Baulkau *et al* 2007) reported that between half and two-thirds of all adults in the world (excluding the USA) were overweight (Body Mass Index (BMI) above 25) or obese (BMI above 30) in 2005. In the USA, once believed to be the world frontrunner in obesity prevalence, the figures are broadly similar. Moreover, the trend is generally upwards and will impact negatively on global health everywhere. Obesity is a risk factor for a range of diseases, including diabetes, circulatory and orthopaedic disorders, and its impact on the future demand for healthcare is likely to be enormous. Obesity prevention has therefore become one of the top public health priorities in many countries.

The aetiology of obesity is complex and includes genetic, environmental and lifestyle factors. In terms of its physiological mechanism, it is a manifestation of an imbalance of the energy equation – excessive caloric intake versus inadequate physical exercise – and those two factors tend to be the focus of public health countermeasures. Changing the dietary and exercise patterns of populations is extremely problematic and requires the implementation of a wide range of behavioural and environmental interventions. Many of these are probably most effectively deployed in early childhood when dietary and exercise patterns are becoming firmly established. A particular cause for concern in many countries is that obesity prevalence seems to be rising faster than overweight prevalence in children in recent years. Regular exercise, either at school or at play, seems to be declining in the lives of many children, partly due to the increased use of computers and other electronic media combined with a growing tendency of parents to transport their children to and from school in cars. Children (and their parents) are bombarded with advertising and marketing of high-calorie food products of dubious nutritional value. Excess caloric intake is, however, only one aspect of poor diet. Even in children of normal weight, a diet overly rich in saturated fat, salt and sugar and deficient in iron, fresh fruits, vegetables and essential fatty acids will have health-damaging effects mediated mainly through poorer growth and brain development.

While obesity and overweight affect almost all countries, we should remember that malnutrition in many parts of the world is still largely a manifestation of extreme poverty and is virtually synonymous with hunger, starvation and death.

Injury

In public health terms, injury is especially noteworthy. Trauma in its various forms remains the leading cause of death and disability in childhood and adolescence, is responsible for a vast amount of pain and suffering, and places a large burden of demand and expenditure on health and other services. Globally, about 10% of all deaths and five (road casualties, self-inflicted trauma, violence, drownings and war) of the 25 leading causes of death are due to injury (Murray and Lopez 1997). Injuries are the leading cause of death in children and young people; they account for 40% of deaths in the age group 10–24 years, which makes up only 10% of the world's population (Patton *et al* 2009). Two related reports published by the WHO recently highlighted the continuing importance of unintentional injuries in children from a European (Sethi *et al* 2008) and a world (Peden *et al* 2004) perspective.

The scale of road traffic injuries (RTIs), and the misery they inflict, is staggering. The GBD study estimated that around 1.3 million people were killed in road traffic crashes (RTCs) in 2004 around the world and up to 50 million were injured or disabled. The highest rates were observed in the African and Eastern Mediterranean regions. Around a fifth of the RTC deaths were in children. Declining trends in these figures have been observed in several developed countries but global RTC injuries are predicted to rise. Within the next decade or two, they are expected to become the fifth leading cause of death worldwide and the seventh leading cause of DALYs lost (Mathers and Loncar 2005).

The global economic impact of road casualties is massive, amounting to an estimated US$518 billion per annum (Jacobs *et al* 2000). Children and young people are disproportionately affected by RTCs, which make them the largest single contributor to childhood injury mortality; over a quarter of a million deaths in the age group 0–19 years were attributed to this cause in 2004. RTI mortality risk increases with age, peaking in the late teenage years, as does the male excess in mortality. More than 90% occur in low- or middle-income countries. About a third of RTI deaths are pedestrians; the remainder are car occupants or two-wheeled vehicle users. The prevalence of long-term consequences, including disability, from RTIs may be around 10 million (or 40 times the annual number of deaths in children from this cause) with pedestrian casualties (around 10% of RTIs) having the poorest prognosis. Post-traumatic stress disorders are common in children following an RTI.

The financial costs of injury are enormous. Though figures are scarce, the direct costs of injury to the NHS in the UK are conservatively estimated at around £2 billion per annum, with global costs to society perhaps 10 times that figure. The costs of child injury care at emergency departments alone in 2008 (Audit Commission/Healthcare Commission 2007) were at least £146 million annually. When older people, especially women, are hospitalised following an injury, the costs are considerably higher due to the longer recovery times, the presence of co-morbidities and the high incidence of complications.

Injury in children and young people is increasingly recognised as the outcome of exposure to a hazardous environment. In Europe, injuries were estimated to be the cause of 23% of all deaths and 19% of DALYS in the age group

0–19 years. These figures dwarf other environmental causes of the disease burden such as air pollution, lead exposure and inadequate sanitation (Valent *et al* 2004). Yet injury prevention, after a temporary renaissance in the last quarter of the 20th century, has been accorded a somewhat lower public health policy profile in recent years, a trend that has generated strong criticism from official UK watchdogs (Audit Commission/Healthcare Commission 2007).

There are many reasons why injury has been neglected. One important one is so obvious that it verges on the banal. The lowly status of injury may be traced to the fragmented way in which various types of injury are reported in official statistics. If all injuries, including road casualties, interpersonal violence, deliberate self-harm and suicide, are combined, their huge impact is immediately apparent. Most reporting systems list all these subtypes separately with the inevitable result that they slide down the league tables of mortality and morbidity. Nevertheless, an attempt to integrate policies relating to both unintentional injury prevention and child protection in England has been launched (Department for Children, Schools and Families 2008) though its status is uncertain in the light of recent political developments in the UK.

Mental illness

Psychological disorders, including alcohol and drug misuse, are extremely common though precise figures are usually unavailable. It is estimated that one in four people will suffer from a mental disorder at some point in their lives. In countries where careful surveys have been conducted, the prevalence of a mental disorder in the population is extremely high and many of these disorders have their origin in childhood or adolescence. In the USA, around 25% of the population meet DSM-IV criteria for annual prevalence (Kessler and Wang 2008). Mental ill health is responsible for substantial mortality (mainly suicides) and morbidity, and accounts for around a third of the total global burden of disability. It is prevalent in all parts of the world but is too often regarded as constituting a low priority in the face of competition for attention from physical diseases. The GBD study places mental disorders on a par with HIV/AIDS in terms of their contribution to total DALYs (Lopez *et al* 2006). In fact, they may well now be the leading cause of disability worldwide. In addition, mental disorders are responsible for enormous social and economic costs in all countries, not least through lost productivity.

Mental disorders may be broadly divided into two types: primary and secondary. Primary disorders are diseases in their own right and include the major psychoses of depression and schizophrenia, as well as dementia and addictions. Depression accounts for around a third of the approximately 450 million people in the world who suffer from mental disorders. If the estimates are to be believed, South Asia seems to suffer a relatively high prevalence of depression while sub-Saharan Africa has a low rate. Women are at higher risk of depression than men. Neurotic illnesses, such as anxiety and phobia, are more numerous and can be equally distressing. Secondary (or associated) psychological disturbance may arise as a consequence of organic disease and trauma and may be even more debilitating than the underlying cause. Examples include some forms of dementia, chronic fatigue, depression and post-traumatic stress disorder.

Many countries, particularly in poorer regions, remain blighted by extremely ignorant, hostile or bigoted cultural attitudes to the mentally ill. People with mental disorders are a vulnerable, neglected and marginalised group that sometimes suffer discrimination, unnecessary incarceration or even maltreatment. Their plight is becoming increasingly recognised. A recent report from the World Health Organization (2010) has highlighted the negative impact of mental illness on population health, wellbeing, educational achievement and productivity, and has called for mental illness in all its manifestations to be included in international development efforts to reduce poverty and stimulate development in poorer countries.

REFERENCES

Audit Commission/Healthcare Commission. *Better Safe Than Sorry – preventing unintentional injury in children.* London: Audit Commission; 2007.

Baulkau B, Deanfield JE, Despres J-P, *et al.* IDEA: a study of waist circumference, cardiovascular disease and diabetes in 168,000 primary care patients in 63 countries. *Circulation.* 2007; **116**: 1942–51.

Beaglehole R, Bonita R. *Public Health at the Crossroads: achievements and prospects.* Cambridge: Cambridge University Press; 1997.

Brhlikova P, Pollock AM, Manners R. Global Burden of Disease estimates of depression – how reliable is the epidemiological evidence? *J R Soc Med.* 2011; **104**: 25–35.

Department for Children, Schools and Families. *Staying Safe: action plan.* Nottingham: DSCF; 2008.

Ehrlich P. *The Population Bomb.* New York: Ballantine Books; 1968.

Fries J. Aging, natural death, and the compression of morbidity. *N Engl J Med.* 1980; **303**:130–5.

Fries JF. Measuring and monitoring success in compressing morbidity. *Ann Intern Med.* 2003; **139**: 455–9.

Garrett L. *Betrayal of Trust: the collapse of global public health.* New York: Hyperion; 2000.

Intergovernmental Panel on Climate Change. *Climate Change 2007 – the science of climate change.* Cambridge: Cambridge University Press; 2007.

Jacobs G, Thomas AA, Astrop A. *Estimating Global Road Fatalities.* Crowthorne: Transport Research Laboratory; 2000.

Kessler RC, Wang PS. The descriptive epidemiology of commonly occurring mental disorders in the United States. *Annu Rev Public Health.* 2008; **29**: 115–29.

Lopez AD, Mathers CD, Ezzati M, *et al. Global Burden of Disease and Risk Factors.* Oxford: Oxford University Press; 2006.

Malthus TR. *An Essay on the Principle of Population.* London: Johnson; 1798.

Mathers C. Epidemiology and world health. In: Holland WW, Olsen J, Florey C du V, editors. *The Development of Modern Epidemiology: personal reports from those who were there.* Oxford: Oxford University Press; 2007. pp.41–60.

Mathers C, Bonita R. Current global health status. In: Beaglehole R, Bonita R, editors. *Global Public Health: a new era.* Oxford: Oxford University Press; 2009.

Mathers C, Loncar D. *Updated Projections of Global Mortality and Burden of Disease, 2002–2030.* Geneva: World Health Organization; 2005.

Mathers CD, Loncar D. Projections of global mortality and burden of disease from 2002 to 2030. *PLoS Med.* 2006; 3(11): e442.

Mathers C, Boerma T, Fat Ma D. *The Global Burden of Disease: 2004 update.* Geneva: World Health Organization; 2008.

McKeown T. *The Role of Medicine: dream, mirage or nemesis?* London: Nuffield Provincial Hospitals Trust; 1976.

McMichael A, Beaglehole R. The global context for public health. In: Beaglehole R, Bonita R, editors. *Global Public Health: a new era.* Oxford: Oxford University Press; 2009.

McMichael AJ, Smith KR, Corvalan CF. The sustainability transition: a new challenge. *Bull World Health Organ.* 2000; 78: 1067.

Mooney G, Irwig L, Leeder S. Priority setting in healthcare: unburdening from the burden of disease. *Aust N Z J Public Health.* 1997; 21: 680–1.

Murray CJL, Lopez AD, editors. *The Global Burden of Disease: a comprehensive assessment of mortality and disability from diseases, injuries and risk factors and projected to 2020.* Global Burden of Disease and Injury Series Vol. 1. Cambridge, MA: Harvard School of Public Health; 1996.

Murray CJL, Lopez AD. Mortality by cause for eight regions of the world: Global Burden of Disease Study. *Lancet.* 1997; 349: 1269–76.

Omran AR. The epidemiologic transition: a theory of the epidemiology of population change. *Millbank Q.* 1971; 83(4): 731–57.

Patton GC, Coffey C, Sawyer SM, *et al.* Global patterns of mortality in young people: a systematic analysis of population health data. *Lancet.* 2009; 374: 881–92.

Peden M, Scurfield R, Sleet D, *et al. World Report on Road Traffic Injury Prevention.* Geneva: World Health Organization; 2004.

Sethi D, Towner, E, Vincenten J, *et al. European Report on Child Injury Prevention.* Copenhagen: World Health Organization; 2008.

Skolnik R. *Essentials of Global Health.* Sudbury, MA: Jones and Bartlett Learning; 2008.

United Nations Environment Programme. *Global Environment Outlook 2000.* London: Earthscan; 1999.

Valent F, Little D, Bertollini R, *et al.* Burden of disease attributable to selected environmental factors and injury among children and adolescents in Europe. *Lancet.* 2004; 363: 2032–9.

World Health Organization. *Global Health Risks: mortality and burden of disease attributable to selected major risks.* Geneva: World Health Organization; 2009.

World Health Organization. *Mental Health and Development: targeting people with mental health conditions as a vulnerable group.* Geneva: World Health Organization; 2010.

World Health Organization. *Global Status Report on Non-Communicable Diseases 2010.* Geneva: World Health Organization; 2011.

Coverage of vital registration of deaths, 2000–2008

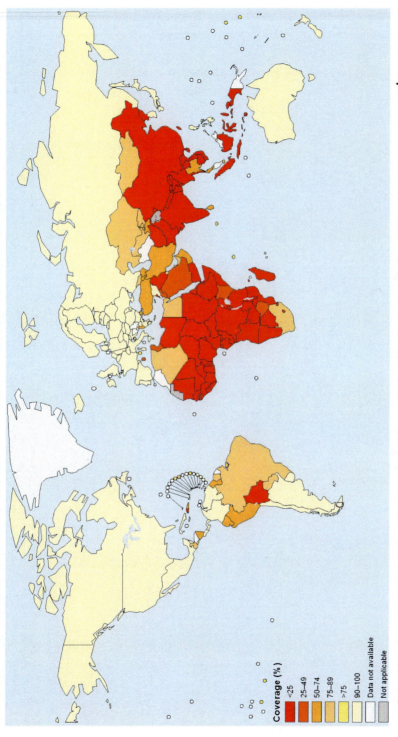

Coverage (%)
- <25
- 25–49
- 50–74
- 75–89
- >75
- 90–100
- Data not available
- Not applicable

The boundaries and names shown and the designations used on this map do not imply the expression of any opinion whatsoever on the part of the World Health Organization concerning the legal status of any country, territory, city or area or of its authorities, or concerning the delimitation of its frontiers or boundaries. Dotted lines on maps represent approximate border lines for which there may not yet be full agreement.

Data Source: World Health Organization
Map Production: Public Health Information
and Geographic Information Systems (GIS)
World Health Organization

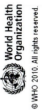

World Health Organization

Figure 1.2 Global pattern of under-reporting of deaths. Source: WHO Global Health Observatory Map Gallery. http://gamapserver.who.int/mapLibrary/app/searchResults.aspx

Age-standardized death rates, 2004

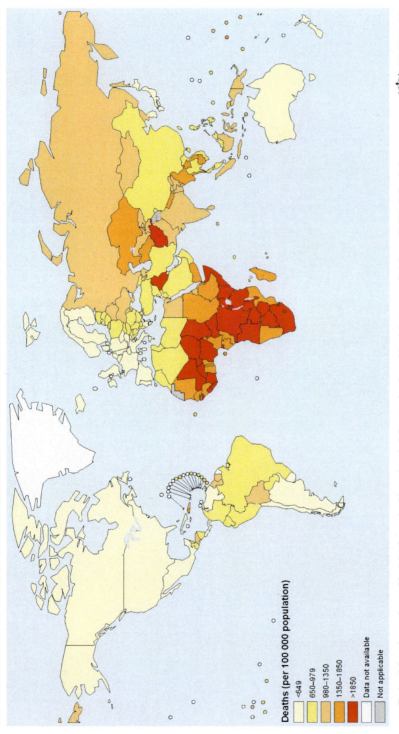

Deaths (per 100 000 population)

- <649
- 650–979
- 980–1350
- 1350–1850
- >1850
- Data not available
- Not applicable

Data Source: World Health Organization
Map Production: Public Health Information
and Geographic Information Systems (GIS)
World Health Organization

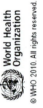

**World Health
Organization**

Figure 2.1 Global pattern of mortality. Source: WHO Global Health Observatory Map Gallery.
http://gamapserver.who.int/mapLibrary/app/searchResults.aspx

Estimated TB incidence rates, by country, 2009

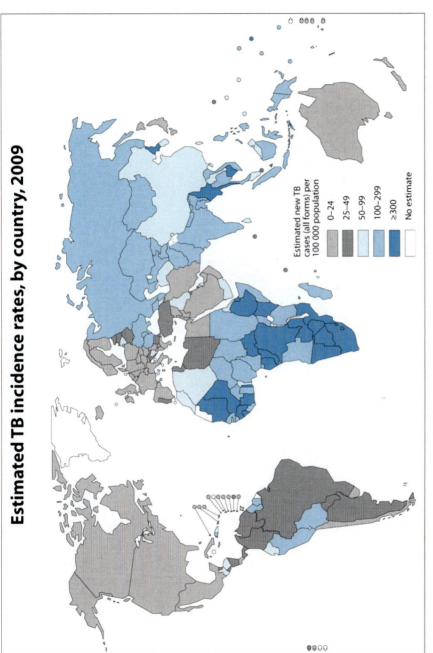

Estimated new TB
cases (all forms) per
100 000 population

- 0–24
- 25–49
- 50–99
- 100–299
- ≥300
- No estimate

Source: *Global Tuberculosis
Control 2010.* WHO, 2010.

The boundaries and names shown and the designations used on this map do not imply
the expression of any opinion whatsoever on the part of the World Health Organization
concerning the legal status of any country, territory, city or area or of its authorities,
or concerning the delimitation of its frontiers or boundaries. Dotted lines on maps
represent approximate border lines for which there may not yet be full agreement.

**World Health
Organization**

Figure 2.3 Global pattern of tuberculosis. Source: World Health Organization. *Global Tuberculosis Control.* Geneva:
World Health Organization; 2010. p.6. http://whqlibdoc.who.int/publications/2010/9789241564069_eng.pdf

Women's deaths from communicable, maternal, perinatal and nutritional conditions as a percentage of total women's deaths, 2004

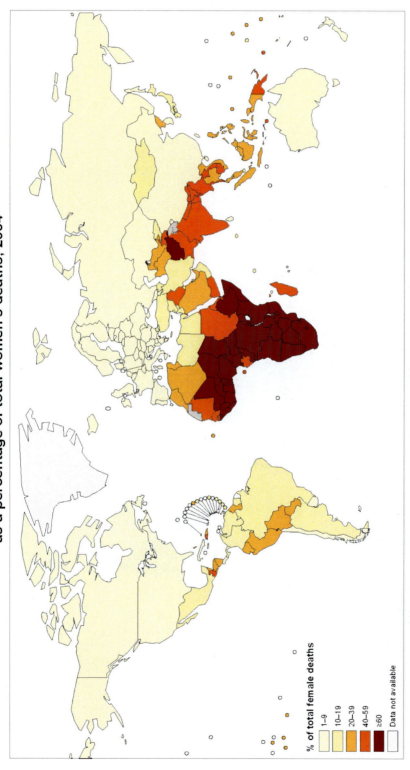

% of total female deaths

- 1–9
- 10–19
- 20–39
- 40–59
- ≥60
- Data not available

The boundaries and names shown and the designations used on this map do not imply the expression of any opinion whatsoever on the part of the World Health Organization concerning the legal status of any country, territory, city or area or of its authorities, or concerning the delimitation of its frontiers or boundaries. Dotted lines on maps represent approximate border lines for which there may not yet be full agreement.

Data Source: World Health Organization
Map Production: Public Health Information
and Geographic Information Systems (GIS)
World Health Organization

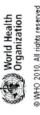
World Health Organization

Figure 3.1 Global pattern of female mortality. Source: WHO Global Health Observatory Map Gallery.
http://gamapserver.who.int/mapLibrary/app/searchResults.aspx

Children aged under five underweight (%), 2000–2009*

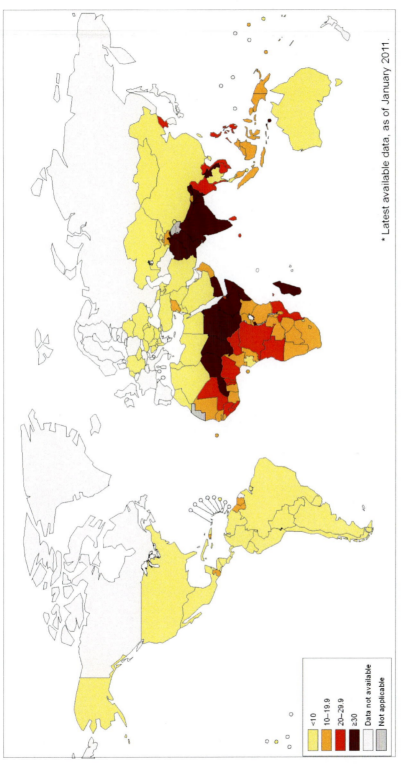

* Latest available data, as of January 2011.

Data Source: World Health Organization
Map Production: Public Health Information
and Geographic Information Systems (GIS)
World Health Organization

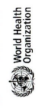

World Health
Organization

Figure 4.1 Global pattern of child malnutrition. Source: WHO Global Health Observatory.
www.who.int/gho/mdg/poverty_hunger/underweight/en/index.html

Legend:
- <10
- 10–19.9
- 20–29.9
- ≥30
- Data not available
- Not applicable

CHAPTER 3

The big one: health inequalities

The experience of health and disease varies enormously between individuals, groups, communities and populations. Mortality and morbidity rates vary across a wide range of intrinsic (internal to individuals) and extrinsic (external to individuals) variables. These variations (sometimes called 'disparities') have long intrigued epidemiologists and social researchers, and have greatly troubled public health professionals.

Health is not only unequally distributed between socioeconomic groups. In the voluminous research literature, health variations have been repeatedly documented across groups defined by ethnicity, gender, geography, educational level and other variables. Some of these (such as education and social class) are inter-related while others are not and may reflect the influence of specific biological, environmental, behavioural or cultural factors. Geographical inequalities within and between countries often reflect underlying socioeconomic variation though other place-specific factors (such as climate, demography and nutrition) may play an independent role. So while the phrase 'inequalities in health' refers to variation in population health status by a wide range of factors, in practice it has been applied predominantly to socioeconomic ('social') ones.

GENDER DIFFERENCES IN HEALTH: BOTH A CAUSE AND AN OUTCOME OF HEALTH INEQUALITY

One type of inequality is so ubiquitous and has such a major impact on global health that it deserves particular attention from the public health community – the plight of women. Gender variation in health is particularly intriguing and relevant to global public health (Skolnik 2008). Despite the fact that men appear to suffer higher mortality and lower life expectancy than women, the intrinsic biological advantage in health that girls and women should enjoy is more than counteracted by the disadvantages and discrimination that they encounter in all parts of the worlds, particularly in regions that are blighted by poverty, poor services, lack of education and geographical isolation.

The determinants of women's health relate to both sex (biological factors) and gender (cultural factors). Biology explains some of the differences: only women suffer cancers of the ovary and uterus, iron deficiency anaemia due to menstruation, and pregnancy-related disorders such as placental bleeding or postpartum infection. There are over half a million maternal deaths each year worldwide and about one in eight of these is thought to be due to unsafe induced abortions. Women seem more susceptible to certain infections including sexually transmitted infections (notably chlamydia, human papilloma virus, syphilis and HIV/AIDS), all of which can lead to serious long-term complications, and to some chronic diseases such as depression and osteoporosis.

Women face the highest risks to their health in the poorest regions of the world, where communicable, maternal, perinatal and nutritional disorders continue to exact a heavy toll on female mortality (Figure 3.1; *see* colour plate section between pages 46 and 47). But the low status accorded to women in many countries places an additional and avoidable burden of illness and risk on their shoulders. The prejudice is so strong in India and China, for example, that many families prenatally identify and then abort female fetuses. Girls may be subjected to the painful and dangerous practice of female genital cutting ('circumcision') that may cause long-term physical and psychological complications without any of the health benefits that may be associated with male circumcision. Female children may be denied food of equal nutritional value as that given to their male siblings, and poor nutrition increases susceptibility to infection. In poor countries especially, much cooking occurs indoors in unventilated spaces and women suffer from the adverse respiratory effects of exposure to open fires and paraffin stoves, as well as from an increased risk of burns and scalds. Women face higher risks of domestic maltreatment, sexual abuse, injuries and violence of all severities often at the hands of domineering male partners. Social and cultural constraints may reduce the access of women to healthcare, education, criminal justice and other services.

All of this has an impact on children who are usually highly dependent on their mothers. In its most extreme form, the death of a mother in childbirth results in her children being neglected and, in some cases, dying as a consequence. And there is increasing recognition of the key influence of women's health on overall family functioning and on the economic performance of a community or country. This insight is reflected in the eight Millennium Development Goals (*see* Chapter 10), six of which have a powerful link to the health, nutrition, education and empowerment of women (Skolnik 2008).

As already mentioned, epidemiologists have long known that men (especially in younger age groups) generally suffer higher mortality and shorter life expectancy than women, at least in developed countries. A European study (White and Cash 2003) reported that most of the premature mortality in men overall was attributable to cardiovascular disease though injury was the largest single cause of death in younger men. The authors urged healthcare practitioners and policy makers to address this important and arguably underestimated source of gender inequality in health.

SOCIAL INEQUALITIES IN HEALTH

Socioeconomic variations in health have been recognised for well over a century. They occur in all regions, countries and communities and are responsible for much debate and soul-searching. Many investigators have sought to document and explain them, while public health practitioners have increasingly committed themselves to address what is widely regarded as an egregious example of social injustice. The two activities – exploring the causes of variations in health, particularly those related to socioeconomic circumstances, and reducing health inequalities – are linked; without understanding the causes of the variations, the task of confronting them is rendered much more difficult. Given the incontrovertible weight of evidence that health inequalities exist and are, in some places, widening, along with the near universal consensus that they need not be inevitable, do we have a coherent explanation as to their causes? With the exception of the most obvious direct effects of extreme poverty and hardship – famine and drought, for example, as causes of starvation and dehydration – the answer is no.

Human beings love single, simple explanations for troubling phenomena. The history of public health is littered with reductionist ('breakthrough') theories that turned out to be wrong. The hardness of drinking water was hailed as the 'cause' of the West of Scotland's high risk of coronary heart disease; consuming too little dietary fibre was thought to explain all manner of chronic disease patterns between and within countries; eating blighted potatoes was believed to place Irish mothers at higher risk of conceiving babies with neural tube defects (anencephaly and spina bifida). To this list of perfectly plausible, if simplistic, theories that turned out to be wrong, in whole or in part, may be added a more dubious set of wholly unscientific assertions about the health inequalities.

In recent years an obsessive focus on politically correct and all-encompassing 'root causes' has emerged. They appear to have evolved from some of the traditional targets of radical polemicists of both the political Left (free market economics, avaricious bankers, neocolonialism, globalisation, international finance, climate change) and the Right (burdensome taxation, mass immigration, excessive legislation, family breakdown, over-reliance on welfare). Some of these ideas probably merely reflect the desire of the mass media to entertain and encourage their audiences. Others have more sinister undertones as they promote, through deliberate or unconscious scapegoating, hostility or worse towards particular sectors, organisations or groups. While these are generally unworthy of serious intellectual attention, we should remain alert to their harmful political consequences.

In attempting to explain social or geographical inequalities in health, Davey Smith and Egger (1996) identified several 'meta-theories of population health': neomaterialist influences, social cohesion and the psychological consequences of inequality, genes, lifestyle factors, and long-term effects of suboptimal early development. They resist endorsing any of these, instead calling for a sustained research effort to unravel the causes of specific diseases. Since their paper was published, new evidence has been presented that has led to vigorous debate about three of these meta-theories: the early biological origins of health and disease, psychosocial factors arising from poverty or income inequality, and the role of parenting and nurturing on emotional development. We will return to these themes in Chapter 4. First, the nature of poverty and its relationship to health deserve closer scrutiny.

The nature of poverty

In the early 19th century, poverty was the norm for all the world's population except for a tiny privileged minority. The huge gaps that have opened up between rich and poor countries since then did not occur by chance. They are entirely the result of relatively small differences in the rates of economic growth that produced a cumulative and dramatic impact over the course of the last two centuries. Britain and parts of its Empire led the way as a result of the Industrial Revolution, followed by Europe and North America. Asia, Africa and Latin America lagged behind and have only recently begun to close the gap.

How widespread is poverty? As always, the numbers depend on definitions. Sachs (2005) distinguishes between three degrees of poverty: extreme (or absolute), moderate and relative. The extremely poor are located exclusively in developing countries and cannot meet the basic needs for survival: sufficient food, water, clothing, shelter, education and access to healthcare. The moderately poor, who live mostly in middle-income countries, can just about meet those basic needs but are permanently perched on the edge of an economic precipice. The relatively poor, who reside in affluent countries, lack access to cultural goods, quality education and other prerequisites for upward social mobility. (Relative poverty is defined in various ways in relation to the norm, such as household income below 50% or 60% of the national median.) Between the moderately poor and the relatively poor is an intermediate category of middle-income households who live mainly in the urban areas of middle-income countries. Numerically, the distribution of these categories across the (approximately) 6 billion inhabitants of the world at the end of the 20th century was as follows:

➤ extremely poor: 1 billion
➤ moderately poor: 1.5 billion
➤ intermediate (neither poor nor affluent): 2.5 billion
➤ affluent (within which are a minority of relatively poor): 1 billion.

World Bank figures indicate that extreme poverty is concentrated in Asia (East and South) and sub-Saharan Africa. This is a dynamic picture with some countries experiencing economic development while others are stagnant. The reasons for this variation are not always easy to discern and simple, single explanations are usually unhelpful. Sachs (2005), in a comprehensive analysis of the global scene, has identified several causes of the failure of economic growth in some of the poorest countries. These are, in order of importance:

➤ low levels of physical, human and natural capital associated with poverty
➤ geographical barriers such as mountainous terrains and transport difficulties
➤ adverse climatic conditions leading to drought, famine and diseases such as malaria, schistosomiasis and dengue fever
➤ the fiscal trap arising from a sparse tax intake from an unproductive population combined with burdensome national debt
➤ corrupt, incompetent or unhelpful governance deterring investment, entrepreneurship and productivity
➤ cultural, religious, ethnic or social barriers to development, particularly in relation to the education of women
➤ geopolitical rivalries leading to protectionist practices, commercial sanctions and sometimes open conflict
➤ lack of innovation due to inadequate funds for investment and a paucity of technological or scientific skills
➤ the demographic trap, whereby poverty leads to higher fertility that exacerbates poverty.

Poverty and disease: a vicious cycle

Poverty and disease are inextricably linked in a bidirectional manner. Poverty is, of course, a key determinant of many forms of ill health though its precise causal mechanism is often complex (except for extreme states of poverty in which the direct impact on health, in terms of lack of shelter, food and clothing, is obvious). The many links between poverty, especially in its extreme form, and illness have been extensively documented. Severe poverty causes malnutrition, high maternal and child mortality, and a low adult life expectancy from a host of diseases, both physical and mental. There are especially close correlations between poverty and injuries, including violence and suicide. Children are peculiarly vulnerable to the health-damaging effects of poverty.

Globally, the diseases that are related closely to poverty are malnutrition in all its forms, diarrhoeal disease, acute respiratory infections, tuberculosis, HIV/ AIDS, and infections of the skin and eyes (Blair *et al* 2010). When countries are compared, there is a clear inverse relationship between gross national product (GNP) and poor health outcomes, particularly infant mortality rates. There are a few exceptions: Sri Lanka and Cuba have low *per capita* GNPs and low infant mortality rates, while Saudi Arabia and Brazil have high GNPs and high infant mortality rates. Generally speaking, and with very few exceptions, poverty is bad for your health.

Reverse causality is also important: ill health can cause and exacerbate poverty. Communities and families that suffer high child mortality rates will try to compensate for these losses through having larger numbers of children and the consequent high fertility rates will trap them in the early stages of the demographic transition (*see* Chapter 2). Children who are constantly ill will miss out on education, fail to achieve qualifications and enter adult life poorly equipped to make a living or contribute to society. Adults with chronic illness or disability may become unemployable and dependent on welfare. A large number of premature deaths through disease robs a society of some of its most productive citizens, thereby impoverishing the country even further. This close and cyclical relationship between poverty and disease is the main rationale for the prominence that public health has received in the framing of the Millennium Development Goals (*see* Chapter 10).

Explanations for effects of poverty on health: income, behaviour and environment

Three fairly clear-cut mechanisms by which absolute poverty impacts on health operate via income, behaviour and environment. Low household income impairs the capacity to purchase adequate nutrition, housing, clothing, heating and other health-enhancing items. Poorer people tend to adopt unhealthy lifestyles such as smoking and excessive alcohol consumption. Living in a deprived neighbourhood places people, especially children, at greater risk of pollution, injuries, low-quality education and a range of other disadvantages arising from an inadequate social and environmental infrastructure. The three mechanisms are closely linked. An inadequate household income will restrict healthier choices, such as the purchasing of nutritious food and warm clothing, and erode the quality of the environment, reflected in hazardous circumstances such as overcrowded housing, dim or absent lighting and absence of safety devices. Unhealthy behaviour, apart from its direct impact on health, will impair employment prospects, reduce household income and contribute to environmental deterioration. And a substandard environment will act as a drain on family resources, thereby reducing income, and reinforce unhealthy, unsafe and risk-taking behaviour.

Whatever the mechanism, poverty damages health and severe poverty damages health severely. Yet absolute poverty, in itself, is an inadequate explanation for the social patterning of health and disease. Relative poverty seems to be just as important as an aetiological factor in ill health. We know this from data that relate to two other aspects of social inequalities in health that are often overlooked. First, a marked social gradient in health occurs in virtually all countries and all communities, including the wealthiest, at all time periods, Japan in the mid-20th century being a possible exception (Mosk and Johansson 1986). Even Sweden, often lauded as a paragon of equality and good public health, has repeatedly documented social gradients in health (Biterman 2007). Second, there is a gradation in the social patterning of health across all social groups in the population rather than simply a contrast between rich and poor. Another way of portraying this is as a stepwise or dose–response relationship between living standards and the risk of ill health. Moreover, there is some evidence that the steeper the social gradient or level of income inequality within a country, the poorer are its national health indicators such as life expectancy or mortality rates. So what is going on?

Wilkinson (2005) discusses three explanations for the consistently reported dose–response ecological (population level) correlation between relative poverty, or social inequality, and ill health: individual income, material circumstances and psychosocial stresses. All probably play their part. The first two are intuitively fairly obvious and have been described earlier; the more money and goods or services a family has at its disposal, the healthier its members are likely to be. The third requires further elaboration.

Indirect effects of poverty on health: unequal societies

In a cogently argued collection of research papers cited in their book *The Spirit Level*, Wilkinson and Pickett (2010) set out evidence in support of an intriguing hypothesis. While acknowledging that poverty, especially in its severest form, is a risk factor for poor health and social outcomes, they contend that it is the degree of income inequality in societies, rather than poverty *per se*, that damages health. They draw their data from two sources: international comparisons of rich countries, and the 50 states of the United States of America. Using a long list of indicators, including life expectancy, rates of obesity, mental illness and homicide, and non-health variables such as children's educational performance, they report a strong and consistent correlation between inequality and outcome, with more equal countries (and states) having better outcomes.

These ecological analyses are highly persuasive in epidemiological terms but cannot reveal the direction of causality or whether an unidentified third (confounding) set of variables (such as intergenerationally transmitted cultural, behavioural or biological factors) are actually responsible for the correlations. This is where the authors propose a plausible, if controversial, possible mechanism: that income inequality has a corrosive and health-damaging psychosocial impact on every social sector within a population. Those in lower social positions, they suggest, feel marginalised, powerless, excluded and resentful, with damaging effects on self-esteem, the nervous and immune systems, behaviour, education and ultimately health. They interpret their data to suggest that the steeper the gradient in social structure, the sharper the psychosocial distress and the worse the health and social outcomes – hence the 'spirit level' metaphor. The practical implication of this mechanism, if true, is profound: adopting polices that merely boost the incomes and material standards of living of poorer families will fail to obliterate social inequalities in health. That is because these inequalities arise from the perceived injustice of the social structure rather than from financial or material hardship *per se*.

This hypothesis is particularly ingenious because it offers explanations both for the inequality–outcome statistical correlations and the social gradients in health and other outcomes, at all levels of relative income. It also has the advantage of securing widespread support from across the political spectrum by undercutting self-interested objections from more affluent families and individuals, who would be asked to make a disproportionate financial sacrifice in the name of income redistribution. The authors suggest that all income groups across the population, not just the poorest, would benefit in health and social terms from their allegedly evidence-based prescription designed to bring about the creation of more equal societies.

Many readers will feel emotionally drawn to these ideas. As a political objective, the creation of a more equal (and hence just, harmonious, productive and healthy) society is hard to resist, and indeed UK politicians of all the mainstream parties appear to have embraced it to a greater or lesser extent. It has, nevertheless, been subjected to strong criticism, from both Right and Left, on several grounds including conceptual woolliness, failure to explore the nature and practicalities of income equality, scientific imprecision, pandering to middle-class angst and political naiveté. Here is a fairly typical example from Hassan (2010).

> *The Spirit Level* yearns for 'evidence based policies', yet, fails to recognise that 'evidence' is never neutral, always about ideas and values. The book's success, itself a tipping point, taps into deep psychological yearnings and liberal guilt about affluence, inequality and the direction of our society in recent years. This is wish-fulfilment and what Isaiah Berlin called the propensity of human beings to want to make the mess of the world into 'symmetrical fantasies'. (Source: Open Democracy, www.opendemocracy-net/ourkingdom/)

All the same, *The Spirit Level's* central hypothesis has received many plaudits and has sparked a fierce controversy, in the UK at least, well beyond the traditional confines of public health. As a clarion call for a more equal and caring society, it has attracted much support. As a treatise based on rigorous scientific investigation, however, its status is much more debatable, with some researchers claiming that the observed correlations are largely a methodological artefact (Jen *et al* 2009). An even more serious objection is that few of their findings cross-refer even obliquely to their recommended economic and political interventions, almost none of which would be regarded as being supported by robust evidence within the scientific community. Their bottom-line prescription, for which their data offer only tenuous support, is explicitly expressed in traditional old-Left anti-consumerist language: 'Further improvements in the quality of life no longer depend on further economic growth: the issue is now community and how we relate to each other'. A contrary view, that stagnant economic growth will lead to rising unemployment, the exacerbation of poverty and consequent poorer health and social outcomes, seems equally plausible. Countries that have prospered economically have achieved their success through consistent economic growth, while the opposite is true of the poorest countries.

Nevertheless, Wilkinson and Pickett have mustered an impressive, albeit selective, array of historical evidence and telling arguments in support of their metaphor. Further research is being undertaken to determine whether the suggested psychosocial mechanisms exist and adequately explain social inequalities in health. As for the epidemiological hypothesis at the heart of *The Spirit Level*, and the economic and political remedies they offer, the jury remains out on both counts.

Previous responses to health inequalities

The health inequalities debate has had a chequered history and has been buffeted by the changing political climate. In the USA, it has tended to focus on racial differences in health, while in the more class-conscious UK, health variation across occupationally defined social sectors has long been the subject of scientific study, though the variable of interest has slowly morphed from 'social class' into 'social deprivation'. While the former attempted to classify individuals according to their specific individual or familial circumstances (often extrapolated from the occupation of the head of the household), the latter is based on a cluster of defined characteristics (such as housing tenure, overcrowding, unemployment, car ownership) that pertain in the place of residence of subgroups of the population. This shift in methodology reflects a change in perception: social status is increasingly regarded as a reflection of where people live rather than who they are.

Around the world, the policy response to the phenomenon has ranged from shoulder-shrugging fatalism to violent revolutionary socialism. Nowadays, few mainstream politicians would argue openly in favour of social inequality. Where opinions diverge is in what should be done about it. If we could eliminate poverty, at least in its most extreme form, we could greatly improve the health of the world's population. Is that a realistic objective? Jeffrey Sachs (2005), a respected American economist, believes we can, given sufficient political will.

Case study: the United Kingdom and health inequalities

There is no shortage of evidence that the health of the UK population varies widely between geographical regions and social groups. In 2009, a report of a parliamentary health committee (House of Commons Health Committee 2009) concluded that: 'Health in the UK is improving, but over the last ten years health inequalities between the social classes have widened – the gap has increased by 4% amongst men, and by 11% amongst women'.

In other words, while some indicators of overall health, such as life expectancy, are improving, socioeconomic inequalities persist or are widening because the health of the poorest section of the population seems to be improving more slowly than that of the most affluent. This is true for all age groups, including children.

The UK is a world leader in the field of health inequalities research and has strongly influenced international thinking in recent decades, culminating in the publication in 2008 of a WHO-sponsored report (Commission on Social Determinants of Health 2008). Social inequalities in health were catapulted to national attention following the publication of the Black Report in 1980 (Townsend and Davidson 1982). That document had been commissioned by the Labour government in 1977 but the manner of its publication, timed to coincide with a public holiday to achieve minimum impact, backfired spectacularly on the Conservative administration of Margaret Thatcher and led to much greater exposure for the report than ministers had intended. The essence of the Black Report was that the health of Britons had generally improved since the foundation of the NHS in 1948 but that the social class gap in health remained and, in some cases, had widened. Black attributed health inequalities primarily to underlying social factors as well as to the negative impact of low income in the poorest families. Subsequent enquiries, including those of Acheson (Department of Health 1998) and Marmot (2010), reached broadly similar if more nuanced conclusions.

The era of political denial about the existence of the problem has passed. It is no longer a matter of dispute between the leading political parties that the health of the poorest section of the British population is improving more slowly than that of the most affluent. The position is well summarised by an extract from an official government statement (Department of Health 2009) that anticipated the publication of the Marmot Review.

> The progress on health inequalities over the last 10 years can be summed up as: much achieved; more to do. The experience against the target makes this clear – there have been improvements in terms of lower rates of infant mortality and longer life expectancy for all groups and areas, but the gap between disadvantaged groups and areas and the rest of the population has remained. The current data (for 2005–07) shows that the gap is no narrower than when the targets were first set ... Health inequalities are persistent, stubborn and difficult to change.

Successive UK governments, along with the devolved administrations of Wales, Scotland and Northern Ireland, have, regardless of the particular political landscape of the day, committed themselves to improving the health of the population, reducing health inequalities and narrowing the gap between the health of the UK people and other comparable populations in Western Europe. Numerous public health White Papers and policy statements are testimony to that. Nevertheless, politicians have had great difficulty in grasping the principle that improving the health of the population will not be secured simply by increasing financial investment in the NHS. The Marmot Review (Marmot 2010) of health inequalities in England stressed the importance of addressing the underlying social determinants of health, foremost among them being poverty and disadvantage.

The Review also highlighted the enormous potential of a lifecourse perspective and emphasised the interaction and synergism between poverty and dysfunctional parenting. Indeed, it stated that 'giving every child the best start in life' was its highest priority recommendation. A related message was that 'upstream' approaches that are applied to short segments of the life cycle (e.g. preventing adults of working age dropping out of employment to rely on incapacity benefit) will have less economic as well as health impact than those targeted at the early years. This strong emphasis on early intervention was bolstered, paradoxically, by the need for public spending cuts. All government expenditure had to be scrutinised, as never before, for 'value for money' and that criterion was invoked by many advocates of early intervention policies (Allen and Smith 2008). Indeed, the Marmot Review argued that the UK 'cannot afford not to address health inequalities', further reinforcing the view of early intervention as a cost-effective investment that will yield future dividends throughout the lifecourse.

The UK experience reflects a recurring theme in the debate about health inequalities that has become prominent in the public health literature: the way that health determinants, health inequalities and the lifecourse all converge in a kind of aetiological nexus. This is the main focus of the next chapter.

REFERENCES

Allen G, Smith ID. *Good Parents, Great Kids, Better Citizens*. London: Centre for Social Justice and Smith Institute; 2008.

Biterman D, editor. Social report 2006. The national report on social conditions in Sweden. *Int J Social Welfare*. 2007; **16**(Suppl 3): 1–240.

Blair M, Stewart-Brown S, Waterston T, *et al. Child Public Health*. 2nd ed. Oxford: Oxford University Press; 2010.

Commission on Social Determinants of Health. *Closing the Gap in a Generation: health equity through action on the social determinants of health*. CSDH Final Report. Geneva: World Health Organization; 2008.

Davey Smith G, Egger M. Commentary: Understanding it all – health, meta-theories, and mortality trends. *BMJ*. 1996; **313**: 1584–5.

Department of Health. *Independent Inquiry into Inequalities in Health*. London: Stationery Office; 1998.

Department of Health. *Tackling Health Inequalities: 10 years on. A review of developments in tackling health inequalities in England over the last 10 years*. London: DH Publications; 2009.

Hassan G. *The fantasyland of 'The Spirit Level' and the limitations of the health and well-being industry*. openDemocracy 2010: www.opendemocracy.net/ourkingdom/gerry-hassan/fantasyland-of-%E2%80%98-spirit-level%E2%80%99-and-limitations-of-health-and-well-being-indu

House of Commons Health Committee. *Health Inequalities. Third Report of Session 2008–2009*. HC 286-1. London: Stationery Office; 2009.

Jen MH, Jones K, Johnston R. Compositional and contextual approaches to the study of health behaviours and outcomes: using multilevel modelling to evaluate Wilkinson's income inequality hypothesis. *Health Place*. 2009; **15**: 198–203.

Marmot M (Chair). *Fair Society, Healthy Lives. A strategic review of health inequalities in England post-2010*. The Marmot Review. London: UCL Institute of Health Equity; 2010. www.instituteofhealthequity.org/projects/fair-society-healthy-lives-the-marmot-review

Mosk C, Johansson S. Income and mortality: evidence from modern Japan. *Population Dev Rev.* 1986; **12**(3): 414–40.

Sachs J. *The End of Poverty*. London: Penguin Books; 2005.

Skolnik R. *Essentials of Global Health*. Sudbury, MA: Jones and Bartlett Learning; 2008.

Townsend P, Davidson N. *Inequalities in Health: the Black Report*. Harmondsworth: Penguin; 1982.

White A, Cash K. The state of men's health across Europe. *Men's Health J*. 2003; **2**: 63–5.

Wilkinson R. *The Impact of Inequality: how to make sick societies healthier*. New York: New Press; 2005.

Wilkinson R, Pickett K. *The Spirit Level: why equality is better for everyone*. London: Penguin Books; 2010.

CHAPTER 4

The human life cycle: does it hold the key?

As in so many areas of human endeavour, public health has become superspecialised into fields such as epidemiology, health surveillance, health protection, health improvement and healthcare management. In some countries, a degree of age specialisation is encouraged and cadres of practitioners have been nurtured who deal exclusively with mothers, children or both (maternal and child health), with adolescents, adults or the elderly. Generalism is becoming relatively rare. Because of the perceived need to recruit, train and manage professionals in a manner that meets defined and transparent standards of competence, some fragmentation of public health is inevitable. Unfortunately, it may also damage our capacity to adopt a comprehensive, strategic response to the multiple health problems simultaneously confronting populations.

If we could conceive of a coherent theoretical framework that would help overcome the intellectual challenges of complexity and fragmentation, and simultaneously offer a strategic platform for public health action, that would represent a great leap forward. One such framework has begun to emerge from the work of epidemiologists over the last few decades. It is best described as the life cycle or lifecourse approach whereby the human lifespan, from conception to death, is viewed as a seamless and dynamic whole. The lifecourse approach has both theoretical and practical attractions. It might just hold the double key for which the international public health community is searching – to making the right 'diagnosis' and implementing the appropriate 'treatment'. A strong early impetus for lifecourse thinking was the realisation that the roots of adult health and illness might originate in early childhood or even in pregnancy.

The insights generated by the work of Barker (Barker and Osmond 1986), Felitti *et al* (1998) and others have refocused attention on the biological and psychological relationships between different parts of the life cycle, from the preconception period to adulthood. This work has major implications both for hypothesis generation in relation to health inequalities (*see* Chapter 3) and for health improvement in all age groups. We can now confidently assert that health and disease (including emotional ill health and antisocial behaviour) in adolescents, young adults and the elderly frequently have their origins in early life (Graham and Power 2004). While that insight is crucial to our intellectual appreciation of health determinants, its practical consequences have been disappointing. The global public health community has been slow to adopt a lifecourse approach in its fullest sense. Nevertheless, the crucial importance of children as a focus for public health strategies aimed at improving the health of the whole population is now widely acknowledged.

CHILDREN ARE THE ADULTS OF THE FUTURE

A particularly unfortunate, though unintended, consequence of a piecemeal approach to public health has been the frequent marginalisation of children. With few exceptions, public health agencies and practitioners in industrialised countries have lately tended to direct most of their attention and resources at the chronic diseases of the middle and older years of adulthood, perhaps because of the disproportionately heavy burden they place on healthcare and other expenditure. That shortsighted view was not always the norm. Until the mid-20th century, improving maternal and child health was widely regarded as a critical step towards addressing the health needs of the population as a whole. Among the factors that have diverted attention away from children in more affluent countries are the rapidly declining child mortality rates associated with the epidemiological transition, major pharmaceutical, surgical and technological advances in chronic disease healthcare, and the remarkable successes achieved by medical researchers in identifying and controlling chronic disease risk factors in adult life.

The role of epidemiology in driving these trends is worth pondering. Epidemiologists have interpreted plummeting infant and child mortality rates in industrialised countries from the mid-19th century onwards as a reflection of improving child health, though these outcomes were often the result of environmental improvements, such as better housing and sewage, that were not specifically aimed at children. Furthermore, adult health indicators remained stubbornly negative, with persistently high levels of premature death and disability. A growing preoccupation with lifestyle and behaviour in adults (and to a more limited extent in adolescents) led to an expanding research effort to understand the roles of smoking, diet, alcohol and exercise in causing or exacerbating chronic conditions such as cardiovascular disease and cancer. As the 20th century progressed, epidemiologists developed increasingly sophisticated methods, including multivariate analysis, to identify and quantify individual-level risk factors for disease and this generated a vast amount of new knowledge and public health activity. Risk factor control, through primary and secondary prevention (mainly screening), certainly produced impressive benefits, including significant reductions in avoidable cardiovascular mortality, but not all population subgroups benefited equally. Moreover, the prevalence of disability, poor mental health (including addictions) and other 'softer' outcomes relevant to quality of life in all age groups tended to remain high and seemed resistant to a risk factor approach to health improvement. New thinking was obviously needed and epidemiologists obliged.

In the late 20th century, evidence began to accumulate that the origins of many disorders of childhood and adult life could be traced to very early life, especially to the intrauterine and preschool phases of the life cycle. It is now apparent that a complex array of health determinants interacts to affect the health and wellbeing of children in ways that have long-lasting effects. These determinants are biological (including genetic inheritance), behavioural (including parenting practices), environmental (whether physical, social or emotional) and contextual (such as politics, culture and war). All these factors play a role in the growth, development and health of the child as manifested by birthweight, nutrition, physical development, language acquisition, educational performance, emotional outlook, social wellbeing and the incidence of illness.

The theoretical and practical implications of these new insights will be explored later in this chapter. They have certainly not yet been fully grasped by public health practitioners and policy makers. A major obstacle is the lack of public health capacity, in the form of appropriately trained personnel, to perform the necessary work. *Child public health* (as opposed to the more traditional and clinically oriented fields of *community paediatrics* and *maternal and child health*) has not received adequate recognition as a specific and high-status professional specialty, with an associated training programme and career structure, in any part of the world. The case for children as a central, specialised focus for public health activity is not yet, it seems, widely accepted.

SHIFTING ATTENTION AND RESOURCES TO CHILDREN

Children deserve particular attention and advocacy as a vulnerable group with special healthcare and health promotion needs, and largely depend on adults (both those known to them and those with wider societal influence) to act on their behalf. This is no longer a controversial idea. Internationally, recognition of the special case of children is reflected in the widespread support accorded, at least in theory, to the United Nations Convention on the Rights of the Child (Office of the United Nations High Commissioner for Human Rights 1990). The Convention contains a 'non-negotiable' set of standards and obligations that commit all states to treating children with respect for the dignity and worth of each individual regardless of race, colour, gender, language, religion, opinions, origin, wealth, birth status or ability.

Apart from their special status as a vulnerable group, children are increasingly viewed as the possible key to better adult health. But there is much less consensus around the scale of resource reallocation to children, relative to adults, required to achieve health improvements in the population as a whole. The relevance of the Millennium Development Goals to children has already been emphasised. Investing health service and other resources in improving maternal and child health, especially before the age of five, may achieve greater health gain, improved behavioural and educational outcomes, and increased economic productivity than investing resources in later parts of the life cycle (*see* Chapter 8) (Heckman 2008, Sinclair 2007). This is partly due to the greater number of potential years of life at stake and partly because of the more malleable health and psychosocial status of children compared with adults. Whether this theoretical knowledge can be turned into practical and effective programmes of early intervention remains to be seen and much research is currently under way to test this hypothesis. In any case, the emergence of persuasive research evidence is unlikely, on its own, to bring about the policy changes needed. In practice, governments have a habit of investing the lion's share of resources in educational and other services for older children and young adults. Shifting investment 'to the left' of the curve (that is, to young children) is difficult though some national initiatives, such as the Sure Start and Healthy Child programmes for England (Department of Health 2008), are predicated on the assumption that a start has to be made sooner rather than later.

GLOBAL BURDEN OF CHILDHOOD DISEASE

There are about 1.5 billion children in the world, of whom around 85% live in developing countries. Around 10 million children under five die each year (equivalent to 30,000 per day), at least half in sub-Saharan Africa, and most of these deaths are thought to be preventable. A key risk factor for child death is malnutrition (Figure 4.1; *see* colour plate section between pages 46 and 47). As Blair *et al* (2010) point out, a child born in Sierra Leone has an almost one in three chance of dying before the age of five, almost 80 times higher than the risk for a child born in Sweden.

The global burden of disease analysis of children aged 0–14 years reported that the top 10 causes of death in low- and middle-income countries were perinatal conditions, lower respiratory infections, diarrhoeal diseases, malaria, measles, HIV/AIDS, congenital anomalies, whooping cough, tetanus and road traffic injuries (Lopez *et al* 2006). In high-income countries the pattern was different; perinatal conditions topped the list followed by congenital anomalies, injuries and infections. Disability (for which data are sparse) is believed to affect around 170 million (over 10%) children worldwide, of which one in 10 is serious. Only one in 50 disabled children receives any type of assistance that could be described as rehabilitation or special educational provision. The causes of disability are multiple and include sensory, locomotor and psychological disorders.

Goal 4 of the UN Millennium Development Goals is to reduce under-five mortality by two-thirds by 2015. Progress has been disappointing, to say the least. Only 16 of 68 priority countries were on target in 2008 to meet this goal and 12 countries were experiencing worsening rather than improving rates. In considering the slow progress of many poorer regions of the world in reducing child mortality rates, Blair *et al* (2010) are clear where the blame lies: 'These setbacks are largely due to failures in policy and commitment by industrialized nations'.

CHILD HEALTH IN THE UNITED KINGDOM

The health of children and young people has provoked growing concern in the UK for several reasons. In 2007, the United Nations Children's Fund (UNICEF 2007) reported that the UK ranked bottom for six dimensions of child wellbeing out of 21 of the world's most prosperous countries. That sent shockwaves throughout all levels of government as well as the numerous organisations and professionals with responsibilities for children in the country. Since then, awareness of the special predicament of children has been rising. In 2008, a WHO-sponsored study (Currie *et al* 2008) reported that adolescents (11–15 years) in the UK were more likely than children in most other countries in Europe or in North America to rate their health as fair or poor, a finding supported by a study sponsored by the Child Poverty Action Group (Bradshaw and Richardson 2009). This is not merely a reflection of negative subjective self-assessments. UK children seem to experience high rates of a range of disorders, physical and mental, and appear more likely to suffer abuse, neglect or other forms of maltreatment than in other similar countries. The incidence of some avoidable infectious diseases in childhood, such as measles (Muscat *et al* 2009), is higher in the UK than in many other European countries. These findings resonated with a hard-hitting report (UK Children's Commissioners 2008) from the four UK Children's Commissioners, a group of expert officials with 'arm's length' responsibility to promote the views and interests of children and young people. They highlighted the 'unacceptable' numbers of youngsters languishing in poverty, the persistence of health inequalities across Britain, the doubling in obesity prevalence over the past decade, and increasing numbers of children suffering mental health problems due to alcohol and drugs.

An educational inspection report (Ofsted 2008) highlighted concerns about English local councils' performance in addressing the health agenda (especially in relation to obesity, substance misuse, teenage pregnancy and child safety) of the Every Child Matters policy (Department for Education and Skills 2004), with the proportion judged good or outstanding declining from 90% in 2006 to 81% in 2007. A review of Sure Start and similar early intervention and enrichment programmes in England concluded that only modest improvements in health outcomes of the under-fives have occurred despite the investment of almost £11 billion since 1998 (Audit Commission 2010).

OLDER PEOPLE

If this book appears to neglect the needs of adults and older people, that is not the intention. It may be a consequence of the author's deliberate attempt to refocus attention on early life. Arguably, adults from about the age of 18 years onwards are relatively well served by the global public health community. Adult age groups consume a particularly large share of health and welfare resources and they have been subjected to extensive epidemiological and healthcare research. They are more likely to articulate their needs, to present to healthcare systems and to lobby officials for service improvements. It is a common feature of public health priority setting that the 'big three' killers of adults – heart disease, stroke and cancer – feature at the top of policy lists with great regularity. Service initiatives to meet the needs of sufferers from chronic diseases such as diabetes, bronchitis, depression and dementia tend to be aimed primarily at older people.

Older people are perceived as important for other reasons too. During working life they are the main source of productivity in a society. In democracies, they are able to exert their influence through the ballot box, by participating in advocacy groups and via the media. By contrast, children and adolescents are relatively powerless, unobtrusive and easily overlooked despite their huge importance to the health of the population as a whole. Nevertheless, the needs of the adult and elderly population deserve serious and proportionate attention. In poorer countries and communities, too many die prematurely or suffer from diseases and disorders that inflict avoidable suffering on both victims and their families, including young children. With increasing life expectancy in all parts of the world, illness and disability loom progressively larger in middle age and towards the end of life with all that that entails for the quality of life of older people and that of their families. And in the future, the later stages of the demographic shift will result in an increase in the total number of deaths, particularly from cancer and injuries, even if age-specific mortality rates fall. Because of the correlation of age with morbidity and disability, it will also inevitably result in the consumption of progressively more healthcare and welfare resources. The corollary of that rather sombre picture is that adults and older people have the potential and capacity to enrich the lives of younger generations, through high-quality parenting and lifelong nurturing, in ways that have major and long-term implications for health. And their experience, knowledge, economic productivity and political influence are potentially invaluable resources for facilitating the kind of public health problem solving that humanity so urgently requires.

LINKAGES ACROSS THE LIFE CYCLE

For most readers of this book, the assertion that child and adult health are linked will be axiomatic. In terms of disease causation or risk, it is almost impossible to consider one without reference to the other. That was widely recognised by the pioneers of public health in the 19th and 20th centuries who expended much effort on establishing health and welfare services for children, often combined with maternity services. Infant mortality was the benchmark, the 'canary in the mine', for the state of health of the population as a whole. If mothers and infants were patently at risk, so were we all – children, adults, the elderly – from the cradle to the grave. For reasons that were touched upon earlier, that conviction was lost or became diluted in many countries as the centrality of maternal and child health in the totality of public health became an increasingly unfashionable concept. In our own time, however, and after many years of stagnation, the research agenda addressing the links between various stages of the lifecourse, and particularly between child and adult health, has been reignited by a diverse series of studies emanating from different starting points.

THE LIFECOURSE, POVERTY AND THREE RESEARCH PARADIGMS

Psychologists, biologists, paediatricians, child psychiatrists and psychotherapists have long been interested in the human lifecourse as a continuous developmental stream as opposed to a series of discrete stages in the life cycle. In the closing years of the 20th century, epidemiologists rediscovered the advantages of adopting a lifecourse perspective on the health of the whole population.

Blair *et al* (2010), in surveying the literature, identified three main research paradigms that are used to investigate the lifecourse: biological influences, psychosocial development and social inequalities in health. All three are closely interconnected and no single paradigm is currently dominant. They share two important principles: that all parts of the lifecourse are mutually interdependent, and that the origins of poor health outcomes in later life may be traced to problems in early life. The three paradigms could all equally well be described, therefore, as variants of a single idea: programming. Lucas (1991) defined programming as the process whereby a stimulus or insult at a critical period of development has lasting lifelong effects. Programming may occur at more than one point in development. It may be conceptualised in terms of three types of causal mechanism: biological, psychological and social.

Biological programming (the Barker hypothesis)

A key question about the role of poverty in creating health inequalities relates to time. Does poverty exert its most lethal effect early in the life cycle, or later, or both? The English epidemiologist David Barker (Barker and Osmond 1986), building on earlier work in Norway (Forsdahl 1977), proposed that chronic adult disorders, particularly cardiovascular disease, could be traced aetiologically to early life, including the prenatal period. He demonstrated an association between indicators (such as low birthweight) of intrauterine malnutrition and a range of diseases in later life. Among the various possible mechanisms to explain this finding, the 'thrifty phenotype' is one of the most convincing. It hypothesises that the small offspring of a malnourished and hormonally stressed mother is maladapted to its environment and is thus placed at greater risk of subsequent obesity, diabetes and heart disease.

The Barker hypothesis has been invoked to explain many apparent links between maternal and infant physiology and later adult health outcomes. It refers mainly to biological aspects of the mother–infant interaction and focuses on nutrition in pregnancy and lactation. While acknowledging the role of both genetic inheritance and subsequent exposure to risk factors (including poverty) throughout later life, Barker and his colleagues propose that there are developmental windows or sensitive periods during which human beings are programmed in early life for subsequent health and disease (mainly affecting the cardiovascular system). The central focus of the hypothesis is on the intrauterine nutritional status of the mother and fetus. The key association that provides the strongest supporting evidence is the one consistently observed between low birthweight and adult coronary heart disease. The Barker hypothesis also seeks to explain intergenerational effects of maternal malnutrition via non-genetic processes. The nature of these is unclear but recent research points to the possibility that some intergenerational effects may be explicable by epigenetics, that is, non-mendelian heritable changes in gene expression driven by the environment in prior generations. Epigenetic or sociobiological explanations (Schooling and Leung 2010) could be compatible with both biological programming hypotheses and broader socioeconomic ones.

An important obstacle to undertaking research in this area is the scarcity of datasets that span pregnancy, infancy, childhood and adult life. Where such data exist, the research findings have been mixed though attempts to refute the hypothesis have so far failed. Nevertheless, there have been several strong challenges, both theoretical and empirical, to Barker's work. Birthweight is known to be a poor proxy for maternal nutrition and its presence may reflect genetic or other influences. The biological mechanisms of programming are unclear and the hypothesis arguably lacks specificity relating to critical periods. Confounding variables, such as breastfeeding, smoking and socioeconomic status, may not have been sufficiently excluded (Ben-Shlomo and Davey Smith 1991).

As low birthweight and other manifestations of maternofetal malnutrition are closely correlated with poverty, the role of fetal programming in generating health inequalities in childhood and later life could plausibly be proposed as a crucial link in the causal chain connecting poverty and ill health. That conclusion has implications for intervention, though these are not necessarily directly translatable from the epidemiological studies as the potential for removing or ameliorating damaging intrauterine exposures may be limited. Moreover, the timing of programming effects may be at odds with the optimal timing of preventive interventions. Smoking, for example, may be a more critical exposure (along with its associated social processes) in pregnancy and in adult life than in childhood, yet anti-smoking interventions may be more efficacious if implemented in childhood than at other points in the lifecourse.

Psychological programming (adverse childhood experiences)

To the biologically framed Barker hypothesis of the early origins of disease was later added a psychosocial one (Felitti *et al* 1998). This traces adult physical and mental ill health to adverse childhood experiences (ACEs) that are often associated with dysfunctional parenting and exposure to severe emotional stress in infancy and childhood. According to these American researchers, who investigated retrospectively reported ACEs in 17 000 socioeconomically homogeneous (middle-class) adult subscribers to the Kaiser Permanente health insurance plan, major disturbances in family relationships are liable to damage infant and child mental health in a way that predisposes to poorer physical and mental health (including addictions), and poorer educational and social outcomes in later life (Figure 4.2). As these disturbances are likely to

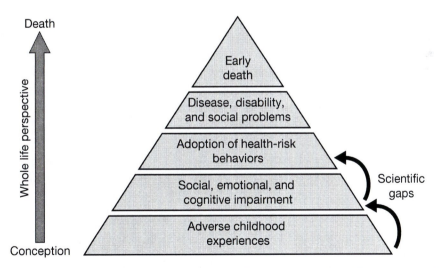

Figure 4.2 Adverse childhood experiences model. Source: reprinted from Felitti VJ, Anda RF, Nordenberg D, *et al.* Relationship of childhood abuse and household dysfunction to many of the leading causes of death in adults: the Adverse Childhood Experiences (ACE) study. *Am J Prev Med.* 1998; **14**: 245–58, with permission from Elsevier.

be more frequent occurrences in socially disadvantaged families, they offer a possible mechanism for the production of poverty-related negative outcomes throughout the lifecourse. Unlike the hypothesis of Wilkinson and Pickett (2010), which implies that health inequalities are caused by the corrosive effect of income inequality on parenting, Felitti *et al* (1998) argue that the reverse occurs – poor social outcomes are the result of poor parenting (although this does not preclude the existence of an intermediate mechanism whereby poverty, inequality, poor health and poor parenting are mutually reinforcing). ACE studies, like those of Wilkinson and Pickett, are retrospective but have an important advantage in that they are supported by intervention studies (Olds *et al* 2007, Sanders *et al* 2003) that suggest a beneficial impact of parenting support programmes on outcomes.

These ideas fit well with recent research indicating the importance of parent–infant bonding, attachment and nurturing in promoting brain maturation and instilling empathic capacity in the developing child. The disruption to healthy emotional development is thus conceived to be a major risk factor for poor mental health, antisocial behaviour and violence. Exacerbating or trigger factors (such as poverty and alcohol) may also play a role in triggering unhealthy behaviours in susceptible (psychologically programmed) individuals. Hosking and Walsh (2005) describe these as 'fuses' that are attached to 'bombs'. Both metaphors are relevant to primary prevention. Some of the fuses may have a similar aetiology to the bombs (e.g. alcohol and aggression) and it is a matter of judgement which should receive priority for preventive intervention.

Felitti and colleagues further argue that the ACE studies appear to validate a central tenet of the early psychoanalytical movement – that early childhood trauma has serious and lifelong effects on later mental and physical health. That Freudian perspective may have diverted attention away from the broader epidemiological significance of this research. The ACE studies demonstrate that high ACE scores are strongly correlated with a range of negative outcomes in adult life, including addictions (alcohol, tobacco, drugs), obesity (a type of addiction), depression, coronary heart disease, chronic bronchitis, violence and suicide.

Critics of the ACE studies have, however, pointed out a number of potentially serious methodological flaws. First, the study data are derived from adult recollections of childhood that may be highly selective, biased and inaccurate. Second, the age range during which ACEs occurred is extremely broad (0–18 years) and sits uneasily with prevailing views of childhood psychological development. Third, the studies were conducted within a particular social and commercial context – a group of relatively affluent American participants in a private health insurance programme. Fourth, an unidentified confounding variable (or set of variables) may have produced spurious associations between ACEs and outcomes.

The researchers have responded robustly to many of these concerns. A retrospective study is, nevertheless, subject to a high risk of bias, confounding and misclassification. There is clearly a need for the study to be replicated elsewhere and for the role of ACEs to be investigated using a prospective (cohort) approach.

If Felitti is right then the implications are far-reaching and are relevant to aetiology, treatment and prevention. If the aetiological pathway is confirmed, it reinforces the case for focusing attention on the early years for a whole range of child, adolescent and adult disorders. And treatment strategies that include an attempt to address and mitigate the ongoing damage caused to the adult by the childhood trauma should be devised and evaluated. Most importantly, primary prevention strategies should seek, through carefully evaluated interventions, to minimise ACEs in the population using whatever tools are available, including parenting support and other early interventions. The methodological challenge for evaluators is formidable, however, as the impact of the interventions may not become fully apparent for several decades.

The corollary of ACEs is nurturing or positive childhood experiences (such as parental affection, stable family structure and non-violent methods of discipline) that could play a health-promoting (salutogenic) role. The impact on positive physical and mental health (and other outcomes) of nurturing as opposed to damaging childhood experiences has been infrequently investigated but appears to be in the expected direction. The salutogenic hypothesis of Antonovsky (1979), whereby resilience and a sense of coherence are acquired by the developing child, and its later elaboration by Eriksson and Lindstrom (2008) are relevant here. Salutogenic processes may be regarded as the mirror images of the pathogenic ones inherent in adverse childhood experiences.

Social programming (socioeconomic inequalities in health)

Socioeconomic influences on health have been well documented even if the precise mechanisms are poorly understood. The social factors that collectively are often labelled 'deprivation' exert their influence, to a greater or lesser extent, on both genders and all age groups in all communities. Individual characteristics or risk factors, such as smoking, poor diet, lack of exercise, low income and adverse childhood circumstances and experiences, only partly explain the socioeconomic correlations with outcomes (through their effects as confounding variables). And place of residence seems to exert a health-damaging effect independently of individual risk factors (Bird *et al* 2010). All of this evidence points to a major ongoing influence of the social environment, regardless of the impact of other variables, on the health of individuals, families and populations.

Given the strong association between poverty in early life and poverty in later life (*see* Chapter 3), the biologically based 'early origins of disease' or fetal programming hypothesis of Barker had to take account of the confounding effects of adult socioeconomic status on infant–adult correlations. Indeed, some critics of the Barker hypothesis produced evidence that social deprivation in later life could explain virtually all of the adverse effects of deprivation in early life (Ben-Shlomo and Davey Smith 1991), though they were at pains to avoid dismissing the importance of early life factors. This led some epidemiologists to argue the case for a lifecourse approach to the investigation of disease aetiology and prevention (Kuh and Ben-Shlomo 1997). Central to this perspective is recognition of the ubiquitous and sustained influence of social factors throughout the lifecourse from conception to death. As in fetal development, there are presumed to be later critical periods when individuals are particularly susceptible to these factors. Because the fetus, infant and young child are in a state of developmental flux, it seems reasonable to assume that social influences exert their greatest impact at these early stages of the lifecourse. If that assumption is correct, this process could be conceptualised as a type of 'social programming'. Social programming could occur, however, at several points along the lifecourse rather than exclusively or predominantly in the early years. Davey Smith (2003) emphasised that generalisations were misleading as specific diseases seemed to have specific aetiologies: stomach cancer, for example, reflects poor social conditions (and consequent *H. pylori* infection) in childhood, high adulthood Body Mass Index (a marker for obesity) is correlated with adverse early life circumstances, independent of later social position (Blane *et al* 1996), while lung cancer was more likely to reflect adult smoking habits. In other words, there is no single, simple answer to the 'earlier' or 'later' question. Both appear to be important. And both may be magnified by the degree of intrapopulation relative inequality, as hypothesised by Wilkinson and Pickett (2010).

If there is a clear potential link between social programming and biological influences, as predicted by the Barker hypotheses, the interaction between both of those models and the psychological one may be less clear but is nevertheless possible. Social inequalities in health start to become evident very early in life, even in pregnancy, and may be mediated, in part, by parental behaviour in relation to nutrition, smoking, drinking and, not least, the quality of the parent–child relationship. Dysfunctional parenting, ranging from an initial lack of empathy and attunement to infants through to outright neglect and abuse, is undoubtedly a cause of poor social and health outcomes later in life. On the other hand, as noted earlier, the causal relationship could operate in the opposite direction, with poverty and social inequalities exerting a corrosive effect on the capacity of parents to nurture their children. It seems likely that both parenting and social circumstances contribute in a major way to the subsequent health and wellbeing of the newborn child (Marmot 2010).

Summary

This is not the place to judge the relative merits or otherwise of the three research paradigms in an attempt to identify one as the pre-eminent model for explaining social inequalities in health. All three appear to have some validity. The various hypotheses and findings should be integrated, as far as possible, into existing knowledge about the early origins of child and adult disease. Ideally, we should develop a single, overarching and coherent theory of health and disease that takes account of both pathogenesis and salutogenesis across the human life cycle. That may prove an elusive goal. What is indisputable is that a lifecourse approach to human health is an extraordinarily powerful tool for investigating both pathogenic and salutogenic processes, and for exploring the nature and origins of social inequalities in health and social outcomes. In particular, the research data, taken as a whole, overwhelmingly support the case for intervening early in life as part of the 'upstream' positioning of health improvement efforts that are 'horizontal' (aimed at multiple outcomes) rather than 'vertical' (aimed at single outcomes) in nature. Public health professionals must now find an appropriate service and policy response to this challenging body of work.

REFERENCES

Antonovsky A. *Health, Stress and Coping*. San Francisco: Jossey-Bass; 1979.

Audit Commission. *Giving Children a Healthy Start*. London: Audit Commission; 2010.

Barker DJP, Osmond C. Infant mortality, childhood nutrition and ischaemic heart disease in England and Wales. *Lancet*. 1986; 1: 1077–81.

Ben-Shlomo Y, Davey Smith G. Deprivation in infancy or in adult life: which is more important for mortality risk? *Lancet*. 1991; **337**: 530–4.

Bird CE, Seeman T, Escarce JJ, *et al*. Neighbourhood socioeconomic status and biological 'wear and tear' in a nationally representative sample of US adults. *J Epidemiol Commun Health*. 2010; **64**: 860–5.

Blair M, Stewart-Brown S, Waterston T, *et al*. *Child Public Health*. 2nd ed. Oxford: Oxford University Press; 2010.

Blane D, Hart CL, Davey Smith G, *et al*. Association of cardiovascular disease risk factors with socioeconomic position during childhood and during adulthood. *BMJ*. 1996; 313: 1434–8.

Bradshaw J, Richardson D. *An Index of Child Well-Being in Europe: child indicators research*. London: Child Poverty Action Group; 2009.

Currie C, Gabhainn SN, Godeau E, *et al*, editors. *Inequalities in Young People's Health: HBSC international report from the 2005/2006 survey*. Copenhagen: World Health Organization Regional Office for Europe; 2008.

Davey Smith G. Introduction: lifecourse approaches to health inequalities. In: Davey Smith G, editor. *Health Inequalities: lifecourse approaches*. Bristol: Policy Press; 2003.

Department for Education and Skills. *Every Child Matters: change for children*. Nottingham: Department for Education and Skills; 2004.

Department of Health. *The Child Health Promotion Programme: pregnancy and the first five years of life.* London: Department of Health; 2008.

Eriksson M, Lindstrom B. A salutogenic interpretation of the Ottawa Charter. *Health Promot Int.* 2008; **23**: 190–9.

Felitti VJ, Anda RF, Nordenberg D, *et al.* Relationship of childhood abuse and household dysfunction to many of the leading causes of death in adults: the Adverse Childhood Experiences (ACE) study. *Am J Prev Med.* 1998; **14**: 245–58.

Forsdahl A. Are poor living conditions in childhood and adolescence an important risk factor for arteriosclerotic disease? *Br J Prev Soc Med.* 1977; **31**: 91–5.

Graham H, Power C. *Childhood Disadvantage and Adult Health: a lifecourse framework.* London: Health Development Agency; 2004.

Heckman JJ. Schools, skills and synapses. *Economic Inquiry.* 2008; **46**(3): 289–324.

Hosking GDC, Walsh IR. *The WAVE Report 2005: violence and what to do about it.* Croydon: WAVE Trust; 2005.

Kuh D, Ben-Shlomo Y, editors. *A Life Course Approach to Chronic Disease Epidemiology.* Oxford: Oxford University Press; 1997.

Lopez AD, Mathers CD, Ezzati M, *et al. Global Burden of Disease and Risk Factors.* New York: Oxford University Press; 2006.

Lucas A. Programming by early nutrition in man. In: *The Childhood Environment and Adult Disease.* CIBA Foundation Symposium 156. Chichester: Wiley; 1991. pp. 38–55.

Marmot M (Chair). *Fair Society, Healthy Lives. A strategic review of health inequalities in England post-2010.* The Marmot Review. London: UCL Institute of Health Equity; 2010. www.instituteofhealthequity.org/projects/fair-society-healthy-lives-the-marmot-review

Muscat M, Bang H, Wohlfahrt J, *et al.* Measles in European epidemiological assessment. *Lancet.* 2009; **373**: 383–9.

Office of the United Nations High Commissioner for Human Rights. *Convention on the Rights of the Child.* Geneva: United Nations; 1990. www2.ohchr.org/english/law/crc.htm

Ofsted. *Annual Performance Assessment (APA) 2007. Report on outcomes.* London: Ofsted; 2008.

Olds DL, Sadler L, Kitzman H. Programs for parents of infants and toddlers: recent evidence from randomised trials. *Child Psychol Psychiatry.* 2007; **48**: 355–91.

Sanders MR, Markie-Dadds C, Turner KMT. Theoretical, scientific and clinical foundations of the Triple P Positive Parenting Programme: a population approach to the promotion of parenting competence. *Parenting Res Pract Monograph.* 2003; **1**: 1–21.

Schooling CM, Leung GM. A socio-biological explanation for social disparities in non-communicable chronic diseases: the product of history? *J Epidemiol Commun Health.* 2010; **64**: 941–9.

Sinclair A. *0–5: how small children make a big difference.* London: Work Foundation; 2007.

UK Children's Commissioners. *Joint Report to the United Nations.* London: UK Children's Commissioners; 2008.

UNICEF. *Child Poverty in Perspective: an overview of child well-being in rich countries.* Innocenti Report Card 7. Florence: Innocenti Research Centre; 2007.

Wilkinson R, Pickett K. *The Spirit Level: why equality is better for everyone.* London: Penguin Books; 2010.

CHAPTER 5

A global public health diagnosis

In earlier chapters, we have seen how the epidemiological data on the state of global public health pose several questions about their interpretation and implications for action. Why is there increasing concern about a possible global health crisis? How can we best summarise the state of global health? What are the reasons for social and other health inequalities? Does lifecourse epidemiology hold the key to better understanding of global health and its challenges? Frustratingly for many readers, I can offer only partial answers to these questions. Yet the very process of posing them, in an informed, evidence-based manner, can prove enlightening and can help us to formulate solutions even if many loose ends remain.

What is the state of global health? We've already explored a large amount of relevant data and sought to place them in a coherent theoretical context. Having interrogated 'the patient' and undertaken a detailed epidemiological examination of the main symptoms and signs, supplemented by a more in-depth investigation of their underlying causes, what conclusions can we reach about the state of global health? What is our provisional global public health diagnosis?

Before proceeding further, it is worth reiterating how a 'public health diagnosis' is arrived at. In essence, it depends on how we use epidemiology, the basic science of public health. There are two components to the use of epidemiology: how we organise the available data and how we interpret them. Although the first may seem technical while the second is judgemental, in reality the two components are closely intertwined.

MAKING A PUBLIC HEALTH DIAGNOSIS

As described earlier, global public health is defined as the application of the public health approach to the health challenges that confront the world as a whole. Its purpose is to enable us to identify, confront and monitor those challenges over time. And the first step in the public health approach (*see* Introduction) is to undertake a needs assessment. That involves profiling, as accurately as we can, the health status of the population in a manner that enhances understanding of both the underlying processes (determinants) and the key health outcomes (burden of disease). All of that is highly dependent on the availability, quality and interpretation of epidemiological data.

We cannot assess the health status of the world's population without collecting, analysing and interpreting global epidemiological data. Too often, we fall at the first hurdle. Researchers have repeatedly complained that estimating the scale and nature of global health is severely constrained by the inadequacy (and often complete absence) of even the most basic demographic and health information. And those data that are available are excessively dependent on the extrapolation of a small number of sample surveys that may too often have serious methodological flaws. Furthermore, the state of the world's health is highly complex and cannot be easily summarised.

Epidemiologists use a range of indicators and techniques to try to describe the health of a population and all have their strengths and weaknesses. The key indicators relate to mortality and morbidity (illness and disability), whether obtained from national statistical agencies or from other sources such as registries and periodic surveys. Healthcare utilisation statistics are among the most widely available though least useful because they are so dependent on the presence or otherwise of supply-side factors such as hospitals, clinics and practitioners.

THE 'PRESENTING SYMPTOMS AND SIGNS'

The significance of an individual patient's complaint to a clinician may be difficult to evaluate. It may signify the presence of serious and possibly lethal underlying disease that demands active and urgent intervention. Alternatively, it may indicate relatively minor or self-limiting pathology that requires no further action. Or it may reflect a generalised, non-specific and non-threatening concern on the part of a patient who is best described as one of the 'worried well'. Distinguishing between these possibilities demands a careful and skilled assessment of the symptoms in the context within which they are offered. The clinician may then undertake a more detailed clinical examination supplemented by further investigation if necessary.

This clinical scenario has parallels with global health. Various experts on the subject have expressed anxieties about the current challenges facing humanity that range from vague unease about the future to predictions of looming and unavoidable catastrophe. Most commentators warn of a lengthening list of daunting population health and related challenges (whether or not they label them 'a crisis') that demand robust and even urgent responses. A minority go much further and predict imminent disaster, including the possible extinction of the human species. A more sober assessment is that we are entering uncharted waters that contain numerous existential dangers. If we ignore them, we may jeopardise the genuine progress in global health that we have made to date. Some of these views are based on a reasoned and plausible analysis of the evidence; others seem rooted in an ideological or philosophical disenchantment with the modern world. All should be assessed in the light of the epidemiological facts, as far as we can determine them.

THE EPIDEMIOLOGICAL 'EXAMINATION'

Putting to one side the more extreme 'complaints' about the allegedly dire state of contemporary global health and the risk of impending catastrophe, what do the epidemiological indicators tell us about the state of global health? There seems to be a mixture of both positive and negative signs, probably in about equal measure (though that is clearly a matter of judgement rather than scientific quantification).

Key initial findings

➤ While the cataclysmic Malthusian predictions have not materialised, the world's continuing population increase undoubtedly poses a serious challenge. Today's population of 7 billion is expected to rise to around 9 billion by 2050, thereafter flattening out. As many countries move through the demographic and epidemiological transitions, they will continue to enjoy improving population health, notably longer life expectancy, in the short and medium term. At the same time, the accompanying combination of falling fertility rates and a rising proportion of elderly people will, in time, be harmful to population health and sustainability.

➤ Along with increasing life expectancy, ongoing nutritional, environmental, technological and healthcare improvements will enhance prospects for a relatively long and high quality of life for most of the earth's population over the coming decades.

➤ Mortality rates have declined more steeply and rapidly in wealthy countries than in poor ones. That reflects widely varying economic development that brings in its wake better environmental and public health infrastructures. The result is that pre-existing health inequalities between countries have widened, as have those within many countries, both rich and poor.

➤ The list of specific, lethal disorders still blighting the world includes alcohol-related disease, unintentional injuries, infections such as HIV/AIDS, malaria, tuberculosis, malnutrition, obesity, chronic disease and mental illness. To these conventional health threats may be added growing fears about the health impact of climate change, environmental damage, civil unrest, human rights abuses, interpersonal violence, terrorism and armed conflict.

Let me add an important caveat to this summary. The generation, analysis and interpretation of all of the above epidemiological data, particularly those relating to international and regional health comparisons and time trends, are seriously hampered by the variability in the completeness, quality, accessibility and reporting of the relevant information.

'FURTHER INVESTIGATION' OF GLOBAL HEALTH SYMPTOMS AND SIGNS

Conceptualising determinants of health and disease

Because the state of global health is impossible to describe in a concise form that does justice to the complexity of its underlying determinants, epidemiologists and other public health analysts have attempted to formulate explanatory pathways, models and other forms of theorising in ways that aid interpretation and action.

A Canadian health minister, Marc Lalonde, was one of the first to explain to the general public that health, disease and disability are outcomes of extremely complex multifaceted processes. He summarised and conceptualised these ideas within a framework that took account of biology, lifestyle, environment and healthcare. Public health experts found the 'health field' model an exceptionally powerful tool for analysis and advocacy. Later, others embellished the concept in various ways in an attempt to introduce a greater degree of both specificity and sophistication (*see* Chapter 1).

The three transitions – and a fourth

To make sense of the changing nature of global health over time, and to respond to it effectively, it is necessary to take account of three interlinked chronological processes that are remarkably consistent across time periods, nations and populations: the demographic, epidemiological and sustainability transitions (*see* Chapter 2).

Poorer regions face a triple burden comprising the old infectious diseases plus the emerging epidemics of chronic non-communicable diseases (including injuries) plus the new health threats associated with globalisation and climate change. This phenomenon is observable not only in the shifting pattern of mortality rates that characterises the epidemiological transition but also in a *risk factor transition* whereby 'affluent' factors such as smoking, alcohol misuse and overweight are increasingly prevalent and impacting negatively on the health of poorer countries.

Poverty, inequalities and global health

All clinicians and public health practitioners are aware of the close relationship between socioeconomic circumstances and the risk of disease. With few exceptions, poverty causes ill health and ill health causes (or exacerbates) poverty. Absolute poverty impacts on health via income, behaviour and environment. Relative poverty is also associated with poorer health, possibly operating via psychosocial mechanisms. These observations are relevant to all countries and communities (*see* Chapter 3).

Extreme poverty is concentrated in Asia (East and South) and sub-Saharan Africa and it is no coincidence that these regions also suffer the worst health in the world. On the other hand, extreme poverty may be found in all regions of the world. Even the most affluent countries contain pockets of severe hardship, as well as relative poverty, and suffer the adverse health effects of social inequalities. And countries that have experienced political turmoil, such as those of the former Soviet Union, have reported sharp upturns in premature mortality in ways that seem unrelated to absolute poverty.

Why some countries have historically experienced sustained economic development and others have not is unclear. As for the future, there are no easy solutions but some senior economists assert that it should be possible to achieve two related objectives by 2025: to end (or at least drastically reduce) extreme poverty and to ensure that all poor countries can progress up the ladder of economic development. The most promising vehicle for achieving these ambitious aims is the commitment of the international community to the Millennium Development Goals.

Lifecourse approach

As we have seen, the origins of many disorders of childhood and adult life can be traced to early life, especially to the intrauterine, infant and preschool phases of the life cycle. Three notable research paradigms have been used to investigate and interpret health-related events across the lifecourse and all may be expressed as programming hypotheses – biological, psychological and social. All three are closely interconnected. Whichever paradigm is favoured at any given moment, the bottom-line message is the same: to understand and improve human health at any age, we have to view health across the entire life cycle, from conception to death, and, additionally, to adopt an intergenerational perspective (*see* Chapter 4). Regardless of the many continuing scientific uncertainties and controversies, a lifecourse approach might just hold the double key for which the international public health community is searching – to making the right 'diagnosis' and implementing the appropriate 'treatment'.

THE BALANCE SHEET OF GLOBAL PUBLIC HEALTH
What are we doing right?

The mixed picture of success and failure in global public health offers fertile territory for both optimists and pessimists. A third attitude – realism – takes account of both the good and bad news. Inevitably, this book may appear more preoccupied with the latter since it has been written to highlight the most serious problems and how they might be solved. But it would be mean-spirited and misleading to ignore the former. And there is no shortage of outstanding examples of public health successes in modern times.

The major successes

The demographic and epidemiological transitions, a feature of affluent countries since about 1800, are now under way in many poorer regions of the globe. Their impact finds statistical expression in steadily improving indices of population health. In recent decades, almost all countries have witnessed major improvements in life expectancy, reduced infant and child mortality, lower fertility, a declining toll of infectious diseases and a growing impact of effective healthcare, both primary and secondary. Two indicators illustrate the sheer scale of progress (Levine 2007). Since 1950, the global death rate in children under five has declined from 148 deaths per 1000 children in 1950 to fewer than 60 deaths per 1000 children by the end of the century. Over the same time scale, average life expectancy in developing countries has risen from 40 to 65 years. And while there is much international comment on the likelihood that the Millennium Development Goal 4 target (67% reduction in under-five deaths between 1990 and 2015) will be missed overall, some countries are actually making excellent progress towards it. For example, China, where nearly one in six of the world's children live, is thought to have achieved the target by 2006 (Rudan *et al* 2010).

Smallpox has been completely eradicated and poliomyelitis may well soon be extinct. Vaccine stocks are high and are increasingly deployed to protect large swathes of the world's population against measles, whooping cough, tuberculosis and many other potentially lethal or debilitating infections. New vaccines against a range of other infections, including malaria and rotavirus, are under development. Effective and relatively cheap therapies for dehydration and bacterial, fungal and parasitic infections have been developed and are being widely disseminated throughout the world, including to its poorest regions. In affluent countries, coronary heart disease prevention and treatment have contributed to improved survival rates and a similar pattern is observable for victims of stroke, severe injury and several forms of cancer, including those afflicting children.

We sometimes forget that these advances have occurred relatively recently in human history. In the words of Bloom (2008):

> If one takes the crudest measure of health, life expectancy at birth – that is whether one is dead or alive at a given age – it is an astonishing fact that half of all the increase in human life expectancy over recorded time occurred in the 20th century. (Reproduced with permission of Jones & Bartlett Learning)

National wealth is not a prerequisite for national health, though it clearly helps. Affluent countries have traversed the demographic and epidemiological transitions with demonstrable benefits accruing to their populations, and many poorer countries have begun, at least, to embark upon them. A large number of international aid programmes, financed by wealthy countries, international agencies, charities and philanthropic donors, are working hard to accelerate the economic development of the poorest countries and are making a discernible impact. There is much cause for celebration here. And we should also recognise the successes that have been achieved by many poor countries or communities through their own efforts to make more effective use of extremely limited resources. What are the key reasons for these successes?

Reasons for past success

Infrastructure

It is never easy to attribute major secular (temporal) trends in health to specific interventions. Some of the improvements in life expectancy across the globe are welcome byproducts of other advances, such as more efficient agricultural technology or the expansion of female education. Others have been achieved by carefully designed and implemented public health measures, in the broadest sense. These include the introduction of clean water, proper sewage management, slum clearance, road safety measures and health-enhancing laws and regulations. Since the Second World War, countries such as the Scandinavian group have led the way by adopting epidemiologically driven, evidence-based public health policies backed by strong professional and political leadership combined with sustained and substantial resource allocation. A sound and well-resourced infrastructure for strategic policy development, implementing interventions and monitoring their impact has been a feature of these high-achieving (in public health terms) affluent countries.

Preventive healthcare

Until the early 20th century, healthcare interventions appear to have contributed relatively little to improvements in population health compared to nutritional and social changes (McKeown 1976). Indeed, epidemiologists have tended to belittle the role of healthcare in improving and protecting public health even when some clinical measures are clearly preventive (such as immunisation and screening delivered within healthcare settings) rather than therapeutic in nature. From the mid-20th century onwards, however, this rather sceptical view of the role of healthcare has undergone a major revision. Epidemiologists now attribute around half of the reductions in cardiovascular disease mortality in North America and Europe to healthcare interventions, including risk factor identification and control, particularly in socially deprived areas (Kiran *et al* 2010).

In the developing world, there have also been spectacular successes as a result of close collaboration between public health and clinical personnel. In 1967, when smallpox was killing close to 2 million victims and infecting many times that number annually, the World Health Organization (WHO) established the Smallpox Eradication Unit and embarked on a programme of mass vaccination combined with disease containment. All regions of the world were included. By 1980, the WHO was able to pronounce the world smallpox free.

Polio eradication has proved more challenging. The WHO launched the Global Polio Eradication Initiative in 1988 when the disease was endemic in 125 countries. Since then, a concerted and well-funded international collaborative effort has led to an estimated 2 billion children being immunised, with the result that only a handful of countries today are affected on any scale by polio. Hope is rising that this lethal and disabling disease will soon be consigned to history.

International programmes

Although malaria remains a massive problem, particularly in Africa, WHO programmes of pesticide spraying combined with antimalarial therapy have achieved impressive reductions in incidence and prevalence in many parts of the world. Trials of a new and inexpensive technology, antimalarial bednets, have yielded encouraging results and should achieve further sustained reductions in malaria incidence in the future.

There are many other notable success stories that demonstrate the way evidence-based, adequately resourced collaboration can make a significant impact. The UNICEF Campaign for Child Survival, launched in 1982, promoted four interventions known as GOBI: growth monitoring of children (to provide early warning signs of malnutrition), oral rehydration therapy (for the treatment of diarrhoea), breastfeeding (to promote healthy growth and prevent infections) and immunisations (against tuberculosis, diphtheria, tetanus, whooping cough, polio and measles). This has contributed to sharp falls in child mortality rates in all parts of the developing world, including Africa. Building on this platform, the Global Alliance for Vaccines and Immunisation was launched in 2000 with a start-up grant of $750 million from the Bill and Melinda Gates Foundation. The target diseases were hepatitis B, *Haemophilus influenzae* type B, yellow fever and several others.

The United Nations Population Fund has, since the 1960s, co-ordinated the dissemination of contraception across the globe, manifested by an increasing uptake from 10–15% of couples in 1970 to 60% by 2000 that has produced close to a halving of total fertility rates. The Fund has helped family planning programmes incorporate a range of other services for women that have improved awareness, literacy and employment, all factors related to declining fertility rates.

Sachs (2005) points to three common themes – technology, leadership and finance – that underpin the success of international health programmes in the developing world. All depend on scaling up and deploying existing knowledge in countries where the need for intervention has been identified. First, appropriate technology should have been developed and shown to be effective in carefully conducted trials. Second, organisational leadership is essential to initiate and co-ordinate efforts involving many agencies and professionals. Third, adequate resources must be injected and sustained to facilitate the achievement of the desired outcomes.

Education

There is a further and often overlooked factor that seems to be an essential ingredient of long-term success in improving the health of poor countries – education. Four developing countries have succeeded in advancing the health of their populations in the face of endemic poverty. These are China, Costa Rica, Cuba and Sri Lanka. Is there a common pattern to these places that might explain their public health accomplishments? They are all very different but in one respect they are comparable: a high priority accorded to education. The case of the southern Indian state of Kerala is highly instructive in this regard.

Kerala is noteworthy for several reasons. First, it has a well-developed primary healthcare system that provides free health services, including family planning, to all its citizens. Second, much emphasis has been placed on nutritional and health promotion programmes aimed especially at mothers and children. A core element has been the strong advocacy of breastfeeding and the regulation of infant foods. Third, the immunisation programme has been run very efficiently. Fourth, the cultural attitude of society towards women has been positive for around a century. Finally, and perhaps most crucially, the state government is fully committed to educating all its citizens to a high level. In 1990, the Ernakulam district of Kerala was declared the first totally literate community in India (Tharakan and Navaneetham 1999). It is probably no coincidence, therefore, that Kerala's health record is so impressive. Infant mortality in the state was 14 per 1000 in 2001 compared with 68 per 1000 in India as a whole, and both the under-five mortality and maternal death rates are equally low. More than 95% of babies are delivered in hospital. In recognition of these achievements, Kerala received the accolade of the world's first 'baby friendly state' from the WHO and UNICEF in 2002.

What are we getting wrong?

The major failures

Against the impressive list of achievements in global health outlined in the previous section must be set several disappointments. Mathers and Bonita (2009) identify three specific groups of continuing concerns: the persistence of health inequalities between and within countries; the fragility of a population's health when challenged by major stressors such as political, social, economic or environmental crises; and the complex mixture of old and new health problems confronting most countries.

A school report on humankind's effort to improve its health might read: 'Making good progress but could do better'. That rather non-committal verdict is widely shared among public health practitioners and policy makers. A minority of commentators would regard the statement as excessively complacent. We need constant reminders that vast numbers of people are still dying or suffering from preventable disorders.

Skolnik (2008) makes this point effectively by citing, from WHO and Global Burden of Disease (GBD) study sources, four disturbing statistics:

➤ 10 000 babies die every day in the world before they are four weeks old
➤ over 500 000 women die in childbirth each year
➤ more than 750 000 children die every year of measles
➤ 1.6 million people die in the world every year of tuberculosis (TB).

These figures, and others like them, are a sobering reminder of the gap between knowledge and its implementation. Yet the numbers themselves may be wrong as the quality of information on global health is so variable. As noted earlier, only a third of the world's population is covered by national vital registration systems, ranging from 95% in Europe to less than 5% in Africa (Mathers *et al* 2005). Where systems are deficient or inadequate, the numbers attributed to specific causes of death have to be estimated by extrapolating from surveys, sample registration systems, verbal autopsies and sheer guesswork. Even greater uncertainty surrounds estimates of morbidity and disability.

Life expectancy at birth has increased in most regions of the world since 1990, with the exception of parts of Africa and the former Soviet Union. In 2004, life expectancy ranged from 79 years in affluent countries to below 50 in Africa – a 60% disparity. Age-specific mortality rates display similar or greater degrees of variation. And the preponderance of avoidable mortality and morbidity in poorer countries has been a recurring theme throughout this book.

A related time trend that suggests serious collective failure is the disappointing decline in under-five mortality. The projected global decline from 1990 to 2015 is 27%, well short of the Millennium Development Goal 4 target of 67% (Murray *et al* 2007). On the other hand, real progress has been made, as a glance at the numbers will confirm: under-five mortality dropped from an estimated 13.5 million deaths in 1980 to 9.7 million in 2005. Moreover, the global average conceals wide variation, including dramatic successes, between countries and regions. This is another example of a mixed picture of good and bad news, the interpretation of which is highly dependent on a combination of the data selected and the mindset of the observer.

Reasons for past failure

If we know so much about the nature, scale and causes of so many global public health problems, and we have already developed numerous potential solutions, why aren't we implementing them? The answer is that we are but our efforts always fall short of the scale of the challenges. We seem to be running to stand still and, in some respects, to be slipping backwards.

We know from history that there is a long lag period between a threat to human health or wellbeing occurring and the mounting of an effective response to it. Often the problem is simply not recognised when it occurs. Social history is replete with examples of what might be described as 'retrospective scandals', including slavery, imperialism, child labour and institutional racism. In the public health field, the list is equally long and includes poor sanitation, slum housing, tobacco and alcohol marketing, drunk driving, hazardous working conditions, inadequate professional training, deficient disease surveillance, poorly administered services and corrupt public governance. Many of these scandals still blight the lives of many people today.

Why is humanity so slow to respond effectively to public health challenges? Good intentions abound but effective action has been limited due to numerous factors only some of which are amenable to change. Listing them all would require a book in itself. Here are just a few.

Paucity of information

There is no question that the inadequacy of public health information systems worldwide has been a major barrier to progress. Here are some of the most serious deficiencies:

➤ the statutory recording of births and deaths is far from universal, with only two-thirds of births and one-third of deaths being properly registered
➤ the quality of diagnostic information on those deaths that are registered is unreliable due to the infrequency of autopsies (physical or verbal), absence of clinical expertise, and cultural or political resistance to some diagnoses
➤ Africa is particularly ill served by national statistical agencies, with only 5% of the African population covered by functioning death registration systems
➤ the development of morbidity and disability measures has been seriously neglected by epidemiologists and information on functional health status is almost non-existent, despite the findings of the GBD studies that around 40% of global lost years of healthy life are due to loss of function
➤ where extensive national health statistics are easily available, they are often hard to interpret due to the absence of analysis and commentary.

When resources are scarce, epidemiological information has too often been regarded as purely a means to an end, a dispensable management tool that, of itself, is less worthy of attention than 'frontline' interventions, particularly. That attitude has frustrated needs assessment, the essential first step of public health without which the development of countermeasures is hampered.

International initiatives such as the GBD study and the monitoring of progress towards meeting the Millennium Development Goals have revealed the size of the health information deficit. Beaglehole and Bonita (1997), writing towards the end of the 20th century, complained that 'little is known about the global burden of disease and even less is known about the global distribution of health'. Little has changed since then despite the sterling efforts of the WHO and other international agencies, working in collaboration with private funders such as the Bill and Melinda Gates Foundation, to improve the quantity and quality of global health information.

Inadequate resources

Although public health interventions are frequently highly cost-effective, resources are always in short supply. In wealthy countries, expensive therapeutic healthcare consumes the vast majority of funds while poorer countries, by definition, lack the economic capacity either to initiate or to sustain public health investment. Carefully directed funding is required to build public health capacity and create a robust infrastructure. The allocation of resources is a political process that may fall victim to ministerial rivalries, incompetence, ignorance, corruption, natural disasters, wars and other unforeseen events. The transfer of resources from richer to poorer countries is a crucial component in tackling global health challenges. The principle has been widely accepted since the Monterrey Consensus in 2002 (United Nations Department for Economic and Social Affairs 2003) when the figure of 0.7% of gross national product was agreed as an achievable target for wealthy countries to transfer to developing countries. Despite this commitment, most countries, including the USA, have failed to meet this modest target. Moreover, assistance has historically been delivered in a highly bureaucratic and inefficient fashion by multiple agencies through development grants, loans, humanitarian aid and a range of specific programmes administered by the UN, the World Bank, the International Monetary Fund and other bodies. All these processes and institutions struggle to achieve progress in the midst of heated public debate, intensive media criticism and a highly politicised, emotionally charged atmosphere.

Lack of leadership, infrastructure and expertise

Effective public health action relies on multiprofessional and intersectoral co-operation both within and between countries. That can cause tensions and rivalries that are best resolved by sensitive but firm leadership. At a strategic level, leadership is often weak due to a perception that public health is 'everyone's responsibility' and that no one department or profession should appear to dominate. Public health policy making is hindered by a paucity of skills, weak advocacy and fragmentation of responsibility between agencies. In poorer countries especially, administrative chaos, neglect of infrastructure, inadequate training and lack of capacity are all commonplace. A further important barrier to progress is the lack of the basic scientific and managerial resources and expertise, particularly in poorer countries, that are so essential to effective action.

The challenge of complexity

In academic circles, much progress has occurred in the intellectual analysis of strategic public health, especially in the realm of conceptual development. This has yet to be translated into effective action. Since Lalonde's health field concept was first expounded, others (notably Evans and Stoddart 1990) have elaborated the theoretical connections between biology, lifestyle, the environment, the economy and politics to the point where we can sum up the position in the phrase 'everything matters' (*see* Chapter 1). That creates an additional problem in that the human brain can cope with only so much theory. Conceptual overload is counterproductive. Superficially, that contradicts the frequent complaint that the public health community is reluctant to acknowledge the sheer scale, complexity and long-term nature of the challenge posed by the poor health record of so many countries and regions. Reductionism is ubiquitous, with almost all of a population's health problems attributed to a single, over-riding cause such as poverty, smoking, alcohol, corruption and conflict. The two phenomena can co-exist: public health practitioners may alternate between a broad-brush approach that addresses multiple factors simultaneously and one that seeks to tackle specific problems sequentially and in isolation. Both approaches, singly or in combination, carry a high chance of failure.

Absence of strategic thinking

At governmental level, policy makers recognise the need to adopt both strategic and tactical measures that take account of overarching political goals while addressing more immediate operational challenges. Comprehensive and integrated public health strategies tend to be non-existent, nebulous or impractical. Policy makers have often been more successful in articulating broad strategic aims or aspirations than in developing vehicles for the practical implementation of interventions over a sustained period of time. A further obstacle is the rather narrow view of health that many policy makers adopt. In a critique of the UK Acheson Report on reducing inequalities in health (Department of Health 1998), Davey Smith *et al* (1998) commended the 39 main policy recommendations but argued that they were weakened by three factors: a lack of prioritisation, by being inadequately concrete and by being uncosted. Above all, they lamented a lack of focus on one central policy – ending poverty, both absolute and relative. And that, they claimed, was achievable through redistributive fiscal measures, increasing child benefits and other forms of family support, and maintaining the real value of state pensions. All these measures lie outside the remit of health ministers yet they are highly relevant to health improvement policy and should therefore feature in any cross-cutting public health strategy.

Excessive individualism

A commonly diagnosed failing of international public health efforts is the alleged failure to adopt a whole-population approach. Part of the problem may be attributed to a tendency to overemphasise individual rather than communal responsibility for health. In the 20th century, epidemiologists focused a great deal of attention on the role of individual risk factors, rather than social or environmental ones, in disease aetiology. This may be reflected in an excessive preoccupation with targeting individuals and families perceived to be 'at risk' of premature mortality through avoidable behaviour or lifestyle choices. Although this attitude is extremely widespread around the world, it seems to be a particular obsession of North America and Western Europe. Public health policy in the UK, for example, according to Lock and Sim (2009), 'has emphasised individual behaviour change and lifestyles, which have been at the centre of its agenda to promote choice in all areas including healthcare provision'.

A related shortcoming has been the excessive focus on individual and familial rather than community or neighbourhood risk. The Alameda County Study (Haan *et al* 1987) demonstrated an area effect on all-cause mortality after taking account of individual socioeconomic position, health practices, social networks and other factors. The Scottish Heart Health Study (Hart *et al* 1997) reported similar findings. The cohesiveness of a community or its 'social capital' may also play a health-protective role, as illustrated by the so-called 'Roseto effect' (Egolf *et al* 1992). There seems to be reluctance on the part of many policy makers to recognise the importance to health of factors that lie beyond the direct control or influence of individuals and families.

High-risk targeting

By contrast, the whole-community or -population perspective, in which an attempt is made to 'shift the curve to the left', has floundered in the political wilderness despite strong evidence of its effectiveness. Rose (1985) and other epidemiologists have demonstrated the 'prevention paradox' that a whole-population, curve-shifting strategy is likely to prove more productive, in terms of overall health gain, than targeting high-risk individuals. A consensus has emerged over the past decade or so that a combination of high-risk targeting and curve-shifting approaches is likely to prove most productive.

An example is the ongoing debate about the balance between universal and targeted home visiting in identifying and supporting dysfunctional families. Despite a growing interest in the formative role of early child development on subsequent health, the natural temptation of public services is to leave the large majority of 'good enough' parents to their own devices and to focus attention on the small minority thought to be at high risk. This strategy is logical but not evidence based. Research has shown that healthcare professionals have great practical difficulty in identifying, in advance, which specific families are likely to prove dysfunctional and thus detrimental to the health and welfare of their children (Wright *et al* 2009).

Neglect of environment

An excessive focus on individual circumstances and behaviour has also blighted informed debate on public health in the media, political circles and even within healthcare professions for the past half-century. This has led to the relative neglect of environmental as opposed to behavioural approaches to health improvement. The phenomenon is a puzzling one given the huge volume of research evidence that environmental influences – physical, emotional, social and economic – play a fundamental role in both pathogenesis and salutogenesis. In part, it may be traced to the health education paradigm that tended to dominate much health promotion thinking in the past. Not only has that approach generated futile attempts to cajole individuals and groups into changing their behaviour, it has also distracted attention from more productive evidence-based, health-enhancing environmental measures. In many countries, this trend has been reinforced by the narrowly defined nature of 'environmental health', a subspecialty of public health that deals almost exclusively with environmental pollution, toxic hazards and the enforcement of environmental standards and regulations.

A further reason for the marginalisation of the environment in public health is political: manipulating the environment rather than encouraging behavioural change is often viewed as paternalistic or intrusive. That prejudice is aggravated by the often ambivalent relationship between policy makers and researchers. The case of alcohol in the UK is instructive. Attempts to curb binge drinking in teenagers by raising its price to consumers have encountered stiff opposition from both the drinks industry and politicians, despite the compelling research evidence that the prevalence of excessive drinking is highly price sensitive. A second example comes from the highly polarised gun control debate in the USA. In some states, the National Rifle Association has sought to outlaw the widespread and evidence-based paediatric practice, aimed at protecting vulnerable children from unintentional gunshot injuries, of asking parents about domestic firearms and their storage.

Silo mentality

In the world of clinical medicine, patients often complain that professionals focus excessively on biological mechanisms rather than the equally important psychological and social factors that make such major contributions to their health and wellbeing. Comparable critiques of public health have suggested the need for greater efforts to break down disciplinary and departmental barriers, incorporate health-promoting as well as disease-preventing activities into public health strategies, and recognise the potentially positive role of healthcare in health improvement. What this amounts to is a call for holism in public health that eschews the traditional 'silo mentality'. It also implies that the public health community should moderate its ideological resistance to clinical or individualistic approaches to health improvement. If healthcare interventions are underestimated or marginalised, a potentially valuable preventive tool may be lost.

Another obstacle to effective public health action has been the tendency to view health and healthcare in predominantly age-specific terms. And just as children should not be viewed in isolation from other age groups, neither can their physical, emotional and social needs be divorced from the context of parents, family, community and society. The complex and interacting factors that comprise these elements continuously influence the developing child and exert long-lasting effects on health and wellbeing. This holistic and ecological (sometimes called the biopsychosocial or socioecological) approach has become a central principle of modern public health. It involves recognition of the role of salutogenic (health-enhancing) as well as pathogenic (disease-producing) influences on the lives of all people. The practical consequence of this approach is that interventions should be planned across the whole lifecourse and be directed at individuals, families and the broader physical, human and psychosocial environment (*see* Chapter 4).

Politicisation of public health

Improving population health requires interventions of a nature and on a scale that will inevitably have political implications. Public health policy is a particularly sensitive area because it impinges on individual autonomy in ways that may seem restrictive or paternalistic. It is also an issue about which everyone seems to hold an opinion that, in open, democratic societies, can be expressed forcefully and sometimes passionately. The result is that much of the public discourse is badly informed, biased and manipulated by special interest groups for commercial or political purposes. Where evidence of the efficacy of an intervention exists, translating research into practice may be difficult in the best of circumstances. In public health, it is especially challenging because many of the proposed interventions are controversial, complex and multifaceted, affect large sections of the populace, involve behavioural or lifestyle changes, require legislation or demand a substantial investment of public funding. The ensuing debate runs the risk of politicisation when key arguments are distorted for partisan reasons. The result is a failure to apply knowledge consistently. Because of this peculiar context, evidence-based policy making and practice have not yet become as commonplace in public health as in clinical medicine.

DIAGNOSTIC SUMMARY: THE STATE OF GLOBAL HEALTH

It is impossible to summarise the current state of global health in a single sentence. We know that we are confronting a mixed picture containing both positive and negative elements. In the last few decades there have been undoubted improvements in global health, notably increasing life expectancy, declining infant and child mortality, and more effective preventive and therapeutic healthcare. But we also need to recognise and respond to what clinicians call the 'red light symptoms and signs' to avoid the balance of global health tipping towards an irreversible downward spiral. Here are some key causes for concern, ranked in no particular order:

➤ the resurgence of old infectious diseases (such as tuberculosis and pneumonia) and the emergence of new ones (e.g. *Cryptosporidium* and *Legionella*) in all countries, but particularly the poorer ones
➤ increasing vulnerability of populations to infection as a result of co-morbidities, microbial resistance to antibiotics and diminishing herd immunity
➤ static or rising maternal mortality rates, after decades of decline, in some affluent countries
➤ plummeting life expectancy in countries of the former Soviet Union since 1990
➤ an increasing and ageing population in the latter stages of the demographic transition
➤ widening social inequalities in health between and within countries
➤ crumbling public health infrastructures in the poorest countries
➤ economic stress arising from macroeconomic economic factors and escalating healthcare costs
➤ environmental degradation, dwindling natural resources and climate change
➤ political instability, corruption and repression
➤ international conflict, civil war and terrorism.

To sum up: the world is facing a long list of serious health problems, many of which appear intractable. More constructively, the state of contemporary global public health may be summarised by two complementary statements.

➤ We have achieved enormous progress in global health in the last half century, notably lower child mortality and improved life expectancy in many countries, but the picture is highly variable, with some large regions of the world showing worrying signs of deteriorating health.

➤ Most of the progress observed up till now may turn out to have been fragile and temporary as a result of newly arising threats from shifting demographic patterns, epidemiological setbacks in the control of both communicable and chronic diseases, global environmental disruption, economic stress, political instability, conflict and several other serious threats.

REFERENCES

Beaglehole R, Bonita R. *Public Health at the Crossroads: achievements and prospects.* Cambridge: Cambridge University Press; 1997.

Bloom BR. Preface. In: Skolnik R. *Essentials of Global Health.* Sudbury, MA: Jones and Bartlett Learning; 2008.

Davey Smith G, Morris J, Shaw M. The Independent Inquiry into Inequalities in Health: a worthy successor to the Black Report? *BMJ.* 1998; **317**: 1465–6.

Department of Health. *Independent Inquiry into Inequalities in Health.* London: Stationery Office; 1998.

Egolf B, Lasker J, Wolf S, Potvin L. The Roseto effect: a 50-year comparison of mortality rates. *Am J Pub Health.* 1992; **82**: 1089–92.

Evans RG, Stoddart GL. Producing health, consuming health care. *Soc Sci Med.* 1990; **31**: 1347–63.

Haan M, Kaplan, GA, Camacho T. Poverty and health. Prospective evidence from the Alameda County Study. *Am J Epidemiol.* 1987; **125**: 989–98.

Hart C, Ecob R, Davey Smith G. People, places and coronary heart disease risk factors: a multilevel analysis of the Scottish Heart Health Study archive. *Soc Sci Med.* 1997; **45**: 893–902.

Kiran T, Hutchings A, Dhalla IA, *et al.* The association between quality of primary care, deprivation and cardiovascular outcomes: a cross-sectional study using data from the UK Quality and Outcomes Framework. *J Epidemiol Commun Health.* 2010; **64**: 927–34.

Levine R. *Case Studies in Global Health: millions saved.* Sudbury, MA: Jones and Bartlett Publishers; 2007.

Lock K, Sim F. Public health in the United Kingdom. In: Beaglehole R, Bonita R, editors. *Global Public Health: a new era.* Oxford: Oxford University Press; 2009. pp.63–83.

Mathers C, Bonita R. Current global health status. In: Beaglehole R, Bonita R, editors. *Global Public Health: a new era.* Oxford: Oxford University Press; 2009.

Mathers CD, Fat Ma D, Inoue M, *et al.* Counting the dead and what they died from: an assessment of the global status of cause of death data. *Bull World Health Organ.* 2005; 83: 171–7.

McKeown T. *The Role of Medicine: dream, mirage or nemesis?* London: Nuffield Provincial Hospitals Trust; 1976.

Murray CJL, Laakso T, Shibuya K, *et al.* Can we achieve Millennium Development Goal 4? New analysis of country trends and forecasts of under 5 mortality to 2015. *Lancet.* 2007; **370**: 1040–54.

Rose G. Sick individuals and sick populations. *Int J Epidemiol.* 1985; **14**: 32–8.

Rudan I, Chan KY, Zhang JSF, *et al.* Causes of deaths in children younger than 5 years in China in 2008. *Lancet.* 2010; **375**: 1083–9.

Sachs J. *The End of Poverty.* London: Penguin Books; 2005.

Skolnik R. *Essentials of Global Health.* Sudbury, MA: Jones and Bartlett Learning; 2008.

Tharakan P, Navaneetham K. *Population Projection and Policy Implications for Education: a discussion with reference to Kerala.* Thiruvananthapuram: Centre for Development Studies; 1999.

United Nations Department for Economic and Social Affairs. *Financing for Development. Monterrey consensus of the International Conference on Financing for Development.* New York: United Nations; 2003.

Wright CM, Jeffrey S, Ross MK, *et al.* Targeting health visitor care: lessons from Starting Well. *Arch Dis Child.* 2009; 94: 23–7.

Section 1 summary

The underlying premise (or, more accurately, hypothesis) of this book is that the world is facing (or is about to face) an acute and potentially disastrous public health crisis that is all the more dangerous for its near invisibility.

To make sense of the changing nature of global health over time, and to respond to it effectively, it is necessary to take account of three phenomena: the demographic, epidemiological and sustainability transitions.

It is no coincidence that the poorest countries suffer the worst health in the world. On the other hand, extreme poverty may be found in all regions of the world. Even the most affluent countries contain pockets of extreme poverty and suffer the adverse health effects of social inequalities. And countries that have experienced political turmoil, such as those of the former Soviet Union, have also suffered upturns in premature mortality in ways that seem unrelated to absolute poverty.

The origins of many disorders of childhood and adult life can be traced to early life, especially to the intrauterine and preschool phases of the life cycle. Three notable research paradigms have been used to investigate the lifecourse: biological influences, psychosocial development and social inequalities in health. All three are closely interconnected.

Whichever paradigm is favoured at any given moment, the bottom-line message is the same: to understand and improve human health at any age, we have to view health across the entire life cycle, from conception to death, and, additionally, to adopt an intergenerational perspective.

We can summarise the position of contemporary global public health in two complementary statements.

➤ We have achieved enormous progress in global health in the last half-century, notably lower child mortality and improved life expectancy in many countries, but the picture is highly variable, with some large regions of the world showing worrying signs of deteriorating health.

➤ Most of the progress observed up till now may turn out to have been fragile and temporary as a result of newly arising threats from shifting demographic patterns, epidemiological setbacks in the control of both communicable and chronic diseases, global environmental disruption, economic stress, political instability, conflict and several other serious threats.

SECTION 2
Treatment

CHAPTER 6

Towards a global public health strategy

WHY WE NEED A STRATEGY

The premise of this book is that global public health, despite its undeniable successes, is either currently facing a crisis or is rapidly heading towards one unless we take evasive action. In previous chapters, the evidence for that premise was presented in a manner that highlighted some of the major problems. Drawing on the clinical analogy, the global health diagnosis highlights a clear cause for concern and the need to prescribe appropriate treatment. In this chapter, we move the debate on to the next stage – intervention (analogous to the treatment plan drawn up by the clinician in conjunction with the patient).

Because the challenge is global, so must be the response. It should comprise a series of measures that are as effective and efficient as possible. These should ideally be incorporated into a global public health strategic action plan. Some of its elements already exist in the texts of international agreements such as the Ottawa Charter of 1986 and the Millennium Declaration of 2000 (along with its associated Millennium Development Goals (MDGs)). Both of those initiatives have been extremely influential in setting the agenda for global public health. But they have their limitations. The Ottawa Charter was a visionary philosophical statement about the nature of health promotion that contained some general exhortations rather than a comprehensive and detailed action plan. The MDGs were more prescriptive and linked to a timeline but their prime purpose was to reduce world poverty, albeit via some explicit public health approaches. The European Union has progressively widened its focus from largely economic and political matters to embrace health-related issues. In 2007, the EU launched a White Paper outlining a European health strategy comprising four principles and three strategic objectives (Commission of the European Communities 2007). These and other international initiatives are all important in their own right and make explicit the visions, values and goals that help motivate public health professionals around the world. In the context of a global public health response, they have not yet been integrated into a single overarching strategic framework.

WHAT IS A STRATEGY?

There is no universally agreed definition of a strategy. The idea derives from military theory though it has been adapted for corporate management purposes to enable organisations to achieve their visions or fulfil their goals.

In essence, a strategy is a plan that indicates how, based on a consideration of the various options, an organisation will get from point A to point B. It can thus act as a statement of intent, supported by proposed action points that together comprise a blueprint or roadmap. Strategy development is closely related to (and often synonymous with) planning and policy making. Theorists argue about whether strategic planning is descriptive or prescriptive, prospective or retrospective, rational (based on logical analysis) or incremental ('muddling through'). Most agree (Idenburg 1993) that, while these debates can be useful, there are really only two essential dimensions to strategic planning: the setting of *goals* (what is the strategy trying to achieve) and the determination of the *process* (how it will be done). Goal setting implies an articulation, in prioritised fashion, of what matters most to an organisation or enterprise. This is the critical initial phase of strategy development from which all else, including the process of implementation, will flow.

An especially helpful definition that reflects all these ideas is that of Schopper *et al* (2006) who defined (for the World Health Organization (WHO)) a policy or strategy as: 'a document that sets out the main principles and defines goals, objectives, prioritised actions and co-ordinated mechanisms'.

COMPONENTS OF A GLOBAL PUBLIC HEALTH STRATEGY

That definition was devised in the context of a specialised purpose or vision (injury prevention) but it is equally applicable to public health as a whole. It makes specific reference to the various components of a strategy, starting with an inspirational and overarching vision (for example, that the world should be a healthier and safer place for all its inhabitants) that is, in turn, predicated on a set of shared values. The vision represents the ultimate destination but getting there requires its elaboration into a set of principles and goals or objectives. The core of a strategy is the enumeration of a list of evidence-based interventions, the effectiveness of which should, following implementation, be subject to evaluation or monitoring. We can build on that list of components to outline the structure of a global public health strategy (Box 6.1).

Identifying a set of shared values on which the global public health community can agree may be far from easy and securing a universal consensus may

---

BOX 6.1 *Components of a global health strategy*

A *global public health strategy* comprises:
➤ shared values
➤ an overarching vision
➤ principles
➤ goals/objectives
➤ actions/interventions
➤ implementation mechanisms/plans
➤ an evaluation framework.

---

prove elusive. Nevertheless, it is surprising how often a majority of stakeholders can be persuaded to unite around a single strategic public health vision. At its heart lies a commitment to human health that is axiomatic. Difficulties may arise in defining or interpreting the concept of health, which may be variously perceived as a state of wellbeing, an aspiration, a basic right, a social value or a resource for everyday living. The underpinning values are likely to be those enshrined in the preambles to international agreements or consensus statements such as the Ottawa Declaration (a particularly good starting point for strategy development). From these, it should be possible to distil a single overarching vision or mission statement, even if it is simply 'to improve global health'. Realising the vision will depend on the articulation of a relatively small number of key strategic principles from which highly focused goals or objectives can be specified. These goals then need to be translated into specific actions or interventions, delivered by appropriate implementation mechanisms and plans. Finally, the impact and outcome of the whole strategy need to be assessed and monitored by means of a robust evaluation framework.

The seven components shown in Box 6.1 are best viewed sequentially although in practice the strategy may evolve in a rather more arbitrary fashion. Subsequent chapters of this book discuss each of the components in greater detail and describe how they can be brought together into a single strategic framework (*see* Appendix). That will, of course, have no official status in that it represents the views of the author alone. Nevertheless, it could offer public health planners some ideas that could be discussed and developed further in the context of 'real-world' global strategy development.

THE STRATEGY DEVELOPMENT PROCESS

Those who work in or with international agencies such as the United Nations (UN) and the WHO are only too well aware of the need for determination, clarity of purpose and enthusiasm to ensure the successful completion of the sometimes fraught process of strategy development. Paradoxically, the best results seem to be achieved when these personal qualities are harnessed to a systematic and analytical approach that sifts the evidence base with a degree of caution and scepticism. In short, strategy development is a highly sophisticated and skilled process.

Two particular aspects of strategy development are worthy of special attention. The first is the endpoint, the final document or statement that sets out the roadmap for producing change. That is self-evidently important as it is the tangible product that will act as the blueprint for implementation. Moreover, as producing a strategy is the *raison d'être* of the exercise, its validity and relevance will be judged (initially at least) on the basis of the content of the document. The second is the process itself. Rather than being merely a means to an end, the process of strategy development contains within it the seeds of the strategy's success or failure. If the process is insufficiently rigorous or clear-sighted, or fails to take account of a wide range of stakeholder perspectives and views, its chances of creating viable, acceptable and effective proposals for action are much diminished.

Schopper *et al* (2006), in offering policy guidelines for national injury and violence prevention, implicitly adopted a rational planning (though non-prescriptive) model that, like their definition of a strategy, is well suited to the development of strategic thinking in global public health. They suggested that policies or strategies should be developed in three overlapping phases:

➤ initiating the process
➤ formulating the strategy or policy
➤ seeking approval.

To these may be added two further headings – devising implementation mechanisms and establishing an evaluation framework.

Phase 1: initiating the strategy development process

The period prior to initiating policy or strategic development may be as important as the process itself. That is because it creates an environment that is generally supportive (or otherwise) of what is being attempted and should help engender a commitment from stakeholders to take action even if its precise nature, at this stage, is unclear.

This initial phase of strategy development comprises four steps that may be pursued either sequentially or simultaneously, depending on circumstances. The steps are:

➤ assess the current situation
➤ raise the level of awareness around the issues
➤ identify leadership and foster political commitment
➤ involve all the key stakeholders.

Assessing the current situation requires the performance of an epidemiological needs assessment using routinely available data on the health status of the world's population, an analysis of existing and potential interventions, a review of the existing policy and strategic environment, and an identification of all the potential stakeholders.

Raising the level of awareness of global health issues includes advocacy by skilled communicators, dissemination of information via the mass media, education of professionals and practitioners in all the relevant fields, lobbying of politicians and opinion formers, and the holding of highly publicised workshops or conferences.

Identifying leadership and fostering political commitment involves working with governments, the private sector, non-governmental organisations (NGOs) and advocacy groups, and ensuring that a lead individual or agency, appropriately resourced, takes responsibility for taking forward and sustaining the process.

Involving the key stakeholders (defined as any person, group or organisation who affects or might be affected by the strategy) requires close consultation and engagement with all the relevant parties, seeking consensus (as far as possible) around the main priorities, and anticipating (and countering) potential sources of resentment, friction, misunderstanding or prejudice.

Phase 2: formulating the strategy

At this point, the strategy itself needs to be articulated in a manner that will achieve maximum impact. This highly skilled task is usually assigned or sub-contracted to a designated individual or to a small group who will work closely with the lead agency and key stakeholders.

The strategy document should be clearly written and well structured so that all the sectors and stakeholders can understand it and how it relates to them. Schopper *et al* (2006) suggest taking three steps in preparing to write such a document:

➤ define a framework
➤ set objectives and select interventions
➤ explain how the strategy will lead to action.

Defining a framework involves setting out, in broad terms, the rationale and mission statement (vision) of the strategy, along with its guiding ethical or operational principles, goals (or objectives) and projected time scale.

Setting goals and/or objectives and selecting interventions involves stating what the strategy is expected to achieve (quantitatively or qualitatively) and how the objectives will be reached through the implementation of specific, evidence-based and practical measures. The difference between goals and objectives is somewhat controversial. For present purposes, goals are general intentions of desired outcomes while objectives are more precise statements of what is expected to be achieved over a defined time scale. Management theorists have advocated the development of SMART objectives, i.e. specific, measurable, action-oriented, realistic and time-specific.

Explaining how the strategy will lead to action includes prioritising the interventions in collaboration with stakeholders, assigning responsibilities, clarifying mechanisms for co-ordination and monitoring, and addressing resource needs.

Phase 3: seeking approval and endorsement

Once the text has been written and revised following stakeholder consultation, the document can then be submitted to the relevant government ministers for approval by their cabinets or leaders, and then, where appropriate, by their parliaments.

This phase has three components, namely:

➤ seeking the approval of stakeholders
➤ securing the endorsement of governments
➤ seeking the support of parliaments.

Seeking the approval of stakeholders may be achieved by holding consultative meetings to discuss the draft document, obtaining feedback on key content, and responding constructively to comments.

Securing the endorsement of governments is a complex task that involves obtaining the approval of officials, ministers and cabinets using whatever internal contacts, organisations or fora may be available within each country.

Seeking the support of parliaments is equally challenging (depending on political circumstances) and may require sustained and determined advocacy, lobbying and media communication.

Once the strategy has been approved, two further essential steps need to be considered – implementation and evaluation – plus the capacity to change in the light of the findings.

DEVISING IMPLEMENTATION PLANS

Public health strategy development is a highly complex process, especially when conducted transnationally. The production of a strategy document is sometimes seen as a worthwhile achievement in its own right and a collective sigh of relief will usually greet its publication. Unfortunately, that is where the trouble may start. Even if the policy is sound and endorsed by all the relevant committees and stakeholders, it may never be implemented. The publication of the strategy is a necessary but insufficient first step. Implementation may be frustrated for many reasons.

There may be inadequate political or stakeholder commitment despite prior declarations of wholehearted support. Interdepartmental disputes may arise as a result of failure to agree on the source of resources (finance, staff or skills) or the prioritisation of interventions. If resources are inadequate and lack ring-fencing, the policy may not progress. Civil servants may struggle to implement the action points if expert advice has been confined to the planning stage. Timing is all-important in the implementation of a strategy. Time scales for the rolling out of interventions should be realistic yet not too protracted. Political time scales may be relatively short term and may clash with the time scales of the strategy. A frequent flaw is the absence of delivery vehicles that specify allocated responsibilities, administrative structures, support staff, reporting mechanisms and time scales. There may be a paucity of intellectual capacity (professional skills, training and research) to ensure effective implementation. Finally, conflicting views about the nature of the necessary monitoring and evaluation procedures can cause the whole enterprise to flounder.

Public health planners may be able to learn from the corporate world, where much thought has been devoted to ensuring that marketing strategies are successfully implemented. The phenomena of strategic 'drift' or 'decay' are liable to occur if staff miss deadlines or lose enthusiasm. For political, financial or other reasons, there may be a relatively short window of opportunity to optimise the impact of a strategy. Gladwell (2000) coined the phrase the 'tipping point' at which a new idea or product seems to seize the public imagination and acquire sufficient momentum to become widely adopted. The corollary is that the strategy may appear to be struggling or moribund until the tipping point is reached.

Lester (1989) suggested seven characteristics of 'best practice' in strategic management, namely:

➤ simultaneous and continuous improvement in the cost and quality of services
➤ breaking down organisational barriers between departments
➤ eliminating layers of management
➤ forging closer relationships with consumers and suppliers
➤ intelligent use of new technology
➤ global awareness
➤ improving human resource skills.

These good practice points may be summarised in three words: efficiency, communication and capacity. The relentless pursuit of all three will optimise the prospects of strategic success. Simultaneously, organisations must remain alert to risks and the opposing forces that could undermine effective implementation. The continuous monitoring of the process and outcomes, in the context of a changing environment, is essential to this function. Strategic implementation should be a flexible, iterative process in which lessons are continuously learned and adjustments made to the strategy itself. In that sense, strategy development and implementation are inseparable and have to progress simultaneously. That means that all organisations that have responsibility for strategic planning and implementation need high-quality information systems operated by staff with the analytical skills that are necessary to help planners make sense of the data. That is why evaluation is so crucial.

ESTABLISHING AN EVALUATION FRAMEWORK

While evaluation may seem to most readers to be self-evidently desirable, lip service is often paid to its inclusion by governments and agencies, and reality frequently fails to match the rhetoric.

Evaluation is usually easier to support in principle than to perform in practice. Problems may arise as a result of terminological confusion. Evaluation undertaken in the context of research is designed to generate knowledge about what can work (*efficacy*); that type of evaluation is different from investigations that assess what does work (*effectiveness*). Synonyms for the latter include monitoring, programme review or audit. All these ideas have been touched upon earlier (*see* Introduction) and will be described in more detail later (*see* Chapter 12). The generally accepted 'gold standard' method for generating evidence arising from research is the meta-analysis or systematic review of randomised controlled trials (RCTs). Lower down the hierarchy of evidence (*see* Chapter 8) are at least one large randomised controlled trial, non-randomised controlled experiments, before-and-after studies and finally expert opinion. RCTs are powerful tools for establishing efficacy (explanatory trials) but these are usually performed in pristine 'laboratory' conditions rather than in the context of 'real-world' programme implementation (pragmatic trials). Normally, strategic planners in the public health field do not have the luxury of distinguishing between different varieties of trials as the evidence base is so limited.

When evaluation is intended to assess the success or otherwise of the effectiveness or efficiency of a strategy (or its components), a rather different methodology is employed. Its purpose is not to generate new scientific knowledge but to guide strategic planners and fine tune the implementation of services or other interventions. In this case, evaluation (or audit) is often conceptualised across the three dimensions of structure, process and outcome (or sometimes 'impact'). These terms are largely self-explanatory but the selection of appropriate measures can be difficult and severely constrained by the accessibility and quality of the available data.

Another popular approach to the evaluation of a strategy is the so-called SWOT (strengths, weaknesses, opportunities and threats) analysis that was developed at the Harvard Business School. Gap analysis is a related concept that seeks to identify and close the gap between the expectation (strategic objective) and the reality (progress achieved to date).

A special kind of evaluation is reserved for population screening. Screening may be advocated for the early identification and avoidance of risk factors, for the detection of signs of disease that require special clinical or social interventions, and for the early diagnosis of potentially debilitating sequelae of disease. Screening is subjected to a specialised type of evaluation because of the unique ethical concerns relating to it (*see* Chapter 12).

FROM GUIDELINES TO STRATEGIES

The guidelines offered by Schopper *et al* (2006) were developed to assist national or regional strategic policy making. At international level, the same principles may be applied, albeit within the context of transnational agencies such as the WHO. That adds several layers of complexity and difficulty. Global strategic planning has to take account of all the relevant factors, both national and international, that could help or hinder the process of policy development and implementation. But the process of strategy development is one thing; the content of the strategy itself is another. The next few chapters demonstrate how the content of a global public health strategy may be developed in a logical, sequential way. The core of the strategy comprises a statement of principles, goals and action points (*see* Appendix). The first step is to decide what constitutes the shared values and ultimate vision of all those involved.

REFERENCES

Commission of the European Communities. *Together for Health: a strategic approach for the EU 2008–13*. Brussels: European Commission; 2007.

Gladwell M. *The Tipping Point*. New York: Little, Brown; 2000.

Idenburg PJ. Four styles of strategy development. *Long Range Plann.* 1993; **26**: 132–7.

Lester R. *Made in America*. Boston: Massachusetts Institute of Technology; 1989.

Schopper D, Lormand J-D, Waxweiler R, editors. *Developing Policies to Prevent Injuries and Violence: guidelines for policy-makers and planners*. Geneva: World Health Organization; 2006.

CHAPTER 7

Values and visions

SHARED VALUES

One of the criticisms of the Ottawa Declaration and other formal international statements on global health is that they are 'top down' because they originate from governments and officials rather than healthcare professionals or ordinary people. (The critics seldom explain what a 'bottom-up' declaration would look like.) What is not disputed is that improving the health and wellbeing of the world's population is a worthy objective that deserves wide and unquestioning support. That gives global public health a tremendous advantage over other international endeavours.

There are various motivating factors for this near-universal support for health improvement. One is that good health is a self-evidently desirable state to which all human beings, in normal circumstances, aspire. Another is that health is a prerequisite for more distal human objectives such as happiness, a high quality of life, economic development and peaceful co-existence. Moreover, most systems of humanitarian or social ethics recognise good health as both worthwhile and attainable. This was not always the case. Graeco-Roman insights, and those of other ancient societies, into public health were largely lost to Europeans in the Middle Ages when a toxic mixture of devout religion and popular superstition swept rationality aside for centuries. The political upheavals in Europe in the 18th and 19th centuries following the French Revolution, combined with the intellectual Enlightenment and the spread of philanthropic social attitudes, paved the way for major reforms aimed at alleviating the plight of the most vulnerable in society, including the poor, the sick and children. Simultaneously, urbanisation and industrialisation proceeded apace with damaging consequences for population health. These were followed rapidly by the launching of ambitious environmental programmes that countered some of these negative trends. They included publicly funded initiatives to demolish slums, build new towns, create new transport infrastructures, pipe clean water to urban residents and dispose of their sewage. Throughout this period, advances in immunology and other biological sciences heralded an era of highly effective mass vaccination against common and lethal infectious diseases.

State intervention, through the provision of large-scale health and welfare services, took off in the early 20th century (often motivated by a concern to improve the alarmingly poor health status of young army recruits) and expanded steadily thereafter. Preventive programmes, initially aimed mainly at promoting the health of mothers and children, and later designed to screen adults for chronic disease risk factors, became an intrinsic part of routine healthcare. Almost all of these public health activities were pursued with a remarkably widespread degree of public and political support.

Most of the public health initiatives of the 19th and early 20th centuries were undertaken at local or national level. The idea of concerted international collaboration in this field was generally confined to a fairly small band of enthusiasts. Following the end of the Second World War, the cause of global health improvement received an enormous boost. Vast swathes of the world had been devastated by the conflict and a daunting humanitarian challenge faced both the victors and the vanquished. Revelations of Nazi atrocities shocked the world into reassessing mechanisms for holding nations to account for the treatment of populations under their control. There was a flurry of discussion on the subject and health was proclaimed to be a fundamental human right, backed by legally enforceable agreements, in all the main international fora.

The preamble to the 1946 Constitution of the World Health Organization (WHO) states that the 'enjoyment of the highest attainable standard of health is one of the fundamental rights of every human being'. This idea was incorporated into the Universal Declaration of Human Rights (Box 7.1) of 1948.

BOX 7.1 *Universal Declaration of Human Rights (1948)*

Article 25 states:
1. Everyone has the right to a standard of living adequate to the health and wellbeing of himself and of his family, including food, clothing, housing and medical care and necessary social services, and the right to security in the event of unemployment, sickness, disability, widowhood, old age or other lack of livelihood in circumstances beyond his control.
2. Motherhood and childhood are entitled to special care and assistance. All children, whether born in or out of wedlock, shall enjoy the same social protection.

In 1989, the Convention of the Rights of the Child asserted that children (below the age of 18 years) have equal rights to adults and are entitled to 'the enjoyment of the highest attainable standard of health and to facilities for the treatment of illness and rehabilitation of health'.

These statements were undoubtedly well-intentioned though cynics might argue that humanitarian concerns, while prominent, were superficial given the undemocratic and oppressive nature of large numbers of governments. The postwar era was notable for an unusual combination of economic austerity, political idealism and a deep hostility on the part of the major Western powers to authoritarian regimes. Governments and leaders around the world were keen to demonstrate their probity and humane credentials to facilitate their inclusion in the newly emerging world political and trade agreements. A relatively cost-free means of enhancing their credibility was to sign up to international declarations on health, human rights and the law. While there may be some truth in that view, it matters little where the underlying impulse for better global health originated. Enlightened self-interest may well have played a part but few will disagree that the impact has been generally beneficial.

Can we identify a collective, consensual vision for today's global public health? There have been many attempts over the years (Box 7.2) and none has succeeded entirely. While a universal consensus is unlikely ever to be achieved, most governments regard public health is relatively non-threatening to their national interests. All idealistic public declarations are liable to be subjected to attack from critics who regard them as too ambitious, too mild or just misguided. In a firm rebuttal of the cynics, Hills and McQueen (2007) offer a vigorous defence of such statements. They suggest that charters, goal statements, mission statements, constitutions and other such documents should be regarded as inspirational rather than specific. Since they often represent the idealised and consequently unattainable goals of the creators, these declarations should not be dismissed as failures but should be recognised for what they are.

At various times, the nations of the world have come together to assert a joint collective vision that is encapsulated by the phrase 'health for all'. The idea

---

BOX 7.2 *World Health Declaration adopted by the world health community at the 51st World Health Assembly, May 1998*

We, the Member States of the World Health Organization (WHO), reaffirm our commitment to the principle enunciated in its Constitution that the enjoyment of the highest attainable standard of health is one of the fundamental rights of every human being; in doing so, we affirm the dignity and worth of every person, and the equal rights, equal duties and shared responsibilities of all for health.

that all of humanity could be free of disease and disability by the year 2000 was espoused by the WHO from the late 1970s (under the charismatic leadership of Halfdan Mahler) in the shape of the Alma-Ata Declaration (World Health Organization 1978) and several subsequent pronouncements. A key element of the Alma-Ata statement (Box 7.3) was the strong advocacy of primary healthcare as a means of improving health, a strategy that was never fully implemented by the signatory countries. Critics variously accused the Declaration of excessive naivety, overdependence on centralised state intervention and undue reliance on unevaluated healthcare approaches to public health challenges. In retrospect, it may have been wildly overambitious and may even have eroded the credibility of the World Health Assembly and the WHO.

The Alma-Ata Declaration was superseded by several other developments. First, the World Bank (1993) published an influential document proposing what became known as 'health sector reform'. It emphasised the need for cost-effectiveness analyses and other hard-headed econometric approaches to public health at a time of economic recession, mounting debts among poor countries and rising healthcare costs. Some commentators welcomed the report's endorsement of public health as an important element in economic development; others claimed that the initiative was an ideologically driven attempt to impose North American and European neoliberal economics on the developing world (Hall and Taylor 2003). While this argument raged, another milestone event, the Ottawa Declaration of 1986 (World Health Organization 1986) (Box 7.4), was making its presence felt. This shifted the emphasis away from health services towards social, environmental and political action and was widely (though far from universally) welcomed as a more pragmatic and valuable exhortation to governments, practitioners and the public than its predecessors.

The Ottawa Charter was an attempt to recapture some of the idealism and ambition of Alma-Ata while recognising the multisectoral and 'horizontal' nature of global public health. That was an innovative idea as several 'vertical' programmes had been launched with fairly narrow objectives, such as reducing child mortality, eradicating polio or tackling the 'big three' infections of HIV/AIDS, malaria and tuberculosis. The Charter was subtitled *the move towards a new public health* and that aspiration was regarded as a key ingredient by its authors, one of whom admitted (Kickbusch 2007) that: 'The aim of health promotion – for us – was to combine a social determinants approach (the old public health) with a commitment to individual and community empowerment (the new public health)'.

A further central component of the Charter was its reformulation of health both as an end in itself (an output) and as a 'resource for living' (an output), prompting Breslow (1999) to hail, perhaps somewhat hyperbolically, the advent of the third public health revolution.

BOX 7.3 *Declaration of Alma-Ata. International Conference on Primary Health Care, Alma-Ata, USSR, 6–12 September 1978*

The International Conference on Primary Health Care, meeting in Alma-Ata this twelfth day of September in the year nineteen hundred and seventy-eight, expressing the need for urgent action by all governments, all health and development workers, and the world community to protect and promote the health of all the people of the world, hereby makes the following Declaration:

I
The Conference strongly reaffirms that health, which is a state of complete physical, mental and social wellbeing, and not merely the absence of disease or infirmity, is a fundamental human right and that the attainment of the highest possible level of health is a most important world-wide social goal whose realization requires the action of many other social and economic sectors in addition to the health sector.

II
The existing gross inequality in the health status of the people particularly between developed and developing countries as well as within countries is politically, socially and economically unacceptable and is, therefore, of common concern to all countries.

III
Economic and social development, based on a New International Economic Order, is of basic importance to the fullest attainment of health for all and to the reduction of the gap between the health status of the developing and developed countries. The promotion and protection of the health of the people is essential to sustained economic and social development and contributes to a better quality of life and to world peace.

IV
The people have the right and duty to participate individually and collectively in the planning and implementation of their health care.

V
Governments have a responsibility for the health of their people which can be fulfilled only by the provision of adequate health and social measures. A main social target of governments, international organizations and the whole world community in the coming decades should be the attainment by all peoples of the world by the year 2000 of a level of health that will permit them to lead a socially and economically productive life. Primary health care is the key to attaining this target as part of development in the spirit of social justice.

BOX 7.4 *The Ottawa Charter for Health Promotion: Ottawa, 21 November 1986*

Health promotion is the process of enabling people to increase control over, and to improve, their health. To reach a state of complete physical, mental and social well-being, an individual or group must be able to identify and to realize aspirations, to satisfy needs, and to change or cope with the environment. Health is, therefore, seen as a resource for everyday life, not the objective of living. Health is a positive concept emphasizing social and personal resources, as well as physical capacities. Therefore, health promotion is not just the responsibility of the health sector, but goes beyond healthy life-styles to well-being.

Prerequisites for Health
The fundamental conditions and resources for health are: peace, shelter, education, food, income, a stable eco-system, sustainable resources, social justice, and equity. Improvement in health requires a secure foundation in these basic prerequisites.

Commitment to Health Promotion
The participants in this Conference pledge:

to move into the arena of healthy public policy, and to advocate a clear political commitment to health and equity in all sectors;

to counteract the pressures towards harmful products, resource depletion, unhealthy living conditions and environments, and bad nutrition; and to focus attention on public health issues such as pollution, occupational hazards, housing and settlements;

to respond to the health gap within and between societies, and to tackle the inequities in health produced by the rules and practices of these societies;

to acknowledge people as the main health resource; to support and enable them to keep themselves, their families and friends healthy through financial and other means, and to accept the community as the essential voice in matters of its health, living conditions and well-being;

to reorient health services and their resources towards the promotion of health; and to share power with other sectors, other disciplines and, most importantly, with people themselves;

to recognize health and its maintenance as a major social investment and challenge; and to address the overall ecological issue of our ways of living.

continued

Five action areas for health promotion are:
Building healthy public policy

Creating supportive environments

Strengthening community action

Developing personal skills

Re-orientating health care services toward prevention of illness and promotion of health.

Three basic strategies for health promotion are to:
Advocate: Health is a resource for social and developmental means, thus the dimensions that affect these factors must be changed to encourage health

Enable: Health equity must be reached where individuals must become empowered to control the determinants that affect their health, such that they are able to reach the highest attainable quality of life

Mediate: Health promotion cannot be achieved by the health sector alone; rather its success will depend on the collaboration of all sectors of government (social, economic, etc.) as well as independent organizations (media, industry, etc.).

Since the Ottawa Charter, there have been several more major international declarations on global health promotion. These were issued from conferences held in Adelaide, Sunsvall, Jakarta, Mexico City and Bangkok. Most were reiterations or expansions of the Ottawa Charter. The Jakarta Declaration (Box 7.5) highlighted the role of partnerships while the Bangkok Charter (Box 7.6) addressed the context of globalisation, climate change and international inequalities.

All these declarations were subjected to intense discussion and lobbying. By their nature, they were the products of compromise to try to meet competing aspirations. Some commentators were unhappy that the negative impact of globalisation was understated, and that public–private partnership was endorsed. Others called for a greater focus on social determinants of health and violations of human rights. Especially strident criticism was voiced by the self-styled People's Health Movement that was established in 2000 by a global network of activists, mainly from developing countries (Chowdhury and Rowson 2000). They sought, through the People's Charter for Health and parallel initiatives, to re-energise the 1978 Alma-Ata principles that had been, according to their world view, marginalised by the liberal (and inevitably iniquitous) market economies of the affluent world, bolstered by the allegedly malign activities

BOX 7.5 *The Jakarta Declaration on Leading Health Promotion into the 21st Century (1997)*

The declaration reiterated the importance of the agreements made in the Ottawa Charter for Health Promotion and added emphasis to certain aspects of health promotion.

The declaration included the following **five priorities for health promotion in the 21st century.**

1 Promote social responsibility for health
2 Increase investments for health development
3 Consolidate and expand partnerships for health
4 Increase community capacity and empower the individual
5 Secure an infrastructure for health promotion

The declaration recognizes that:
➤ Participation is necessary for change
➤ Health literacy is essential for participation and emphasizes the need for access to education and information and hence, the empowerment of individuals and communities.

Combinations of five strategies for health promotion are more effective than single-track approaches:
➤ build healthy public policy
➤ create supportive environments
➤ strengthen community action
➤ develop personal skills
➤ reorientate health services.

BOX 7.6 *The Bangkok Charter for Health Promotion in a Globalized World (2005)*

The Bangkok Charter for Health Promotion in a Globalized World identifies actions, commitments and pledges required to address the determinants of health in a globalized world. It recognizes: the inequality between developed and developing nations, the changing trend of communication and consumption in a globalized world, urbanization, global environmental change, and commercialization.

Required actions
To make further advances in implementing these strategies, all sectors and settings must act to: *continued*

➤ **advocate** for health based on human rights and solidarity
➤ **invest** in sustainable policies, actions and infrastructure to address the determinants of health
➤ **build capacity** for policy development, leadership, health promotion practice, knowledge transfer and research, and health literacy
➤ **regulate and legislate** to ensure a high level of protection from harm and enable equal opportunity for health and well-being for all people
➤ **partner and build alliances** with public, private, nongovernmental and international organizations and civil society to create sustainable actions.

Key commitments
The four key commitments are to make the promotion of health:
➤ central to the global development agenda
➤ a core responsibility for all of government
➤ a key focus of communities and civil society
➤ a requirement for good corporate practice.

Closing the implementation gap
Since the adoption of the Ottawa Charter, a significant number of resolutions at national and global level have been signed in support of health promotion, but these have not always been followed by action. The participants of this Bangkok Conference forcefully call on Member States of the World Health Organization to close this implementation gap and move to policies and partnerships for action.

Call for action
Conference participants request the World Health Organization and its Member States, in collaboration with others, to allocate resources for health promotion, initiate plans of action and monitor performance through appropriate indicators and targets, and to report on progress at regular intervals. United Nations organizations are asked to explore the benefits of developing a Global Treaty for Health.

of the World Bank and the International Monetary Fund. Given the breadth of the global health agenda and the high emotional temperature engendered by these debates, it is hardly surprising that each declaration, however carefully composed, leaves a cluster of disgruntled stakeholders in its wake. What is truly remarkable is that the WHO has been able to secure the extent of agreement that it has.

Where does all this philosophising about values and visions for global health lead us? Perhaps not far enough. Returning to first principles, we can express the key objectives of public health as a vision or mission statement that is not dependent on international public health politics. Public health, as initially advocated by Winslow and later by the UK Faculty of Public Health, is simply about improving health and preventing disease. Its historical roots in the social justice and welfare reform movements of the 19th century have stood it in good stead through the succeeding decades. These idealistic impulses have never withered and have been re-energised by the growing interest in the related objectives of reducing social inequalities in health and preserving the natural environment.

Stirring these various ingredients into the pot, here is one of many possible versions of a global public health mission statement for our time.

> To embrace, at a global level, a form of public health that is holistic in scope and aspires to influence the health of populations with a view to:
> * improving and protecting health and wellbeing (physical, mental and social)
> * preventing ill health (and the risk of ill health), disability and suffering
> * reducing health inequalities between genders, races, social groups, communities and countries
> * nurturing an ecologically sustainable environment for future generations.

That statement avoids divisive political posturing and has the additional advantages of simplicity and concision. It will serve our purpose. The next three chapters will discuss a set of proposed principles, goals and interventions that could constitute a global public health strategy for the 21st century.

REFERENCES

Breslow L. From disease prevention to health promotion. *JAMA*. 1999; **281**: 1030–3.

Chowdhury Z, Rowson M. The people's health assembly. *BMJ*. 2000; **321**: 1361–2.

Hall JJ, Taylor R. Health for all beyond 2000: the demise of the Alma-Ata Declaration and primary health care in developing countries. *Med J Austral*. 2003; **178**: 17–20.

Hills M, McQueen D. At issue: two decades of the Ottawa Charter. *Promot Educ Suppl*. 2007; **2**: 5.

Kickbusch I. The move towards a new public health. *Promot Educ Suppl*. 2007; **2**: 9.

World Bank. *World Development Report 1993: investing in health*. New York: Oxford University Press; 1993.

World Health Organization. *Alma-Ata. Primary Health Care* (Health for All Series No. 1). Geneva: World Health Organization; 1978.

World Health Organization. *Ottawa Charter for Health Promotion*. Geneva: World Health Organization; 1986).

CHAPTER 8

Changing the mindset: five overarching principles

Any reasonably well-informed and thoughtful reader will be able to draw up a short list of some of the measures that might be taken to improve global health. These interventions are potentially extremely wide-ranging and encompass efforts to improve life circumstances, behaviour and outcomes through a combination of primary, secondary and tertiary prevention. They would certainly include poverty reduction and amelioration (especially in the world's poorest regions), better nutrition for mothers and children, increased vaccination rates against common diseases such as measles, polio and tuberculosis, the wider dissemination of antimalarial bed nets, universal road and product safety legislation and enforcement, improved primary and secondary healthcare worldwide, and increased support for families with disabled children and older people.

None of these items is particularly controversial. Each addresses a key health challenge in a rational and evidence-based manner. The problem with the above list is that, as a menu, it fails to add up to a satisfying meal. That is because it has been drawn up in an arbitrary and almost random way, lacking coherence because it seems disconnected from any theoretical perspective, or from a clearly expressed set of underlying values or principles. And this is fairly typical of the discourse around much public health activity today. Public health is never value free even if its practitioners seldom express those values explicitly. That creates a problem on two counts. First, external observers, members of the target population and other key stakeholders will not necessarily know or be able to surmise what the underlying values are. Nature abhors a vacuum and the absence of a statement of values may lead to ill-founded and destructive accusations of a hidden agenda or even a conspiracy. Second, those responsible for planning and delivering a public health programme may have difficulty arguing the case for support to colleagues, fundholders or government officials if the values underpinning the programme are obscure.

The concept of value-driven public health may seem opaque or irrelevant to many public health practitioners. The demands of daily work generally trump philosophical musings. What is needed, then, is a change of collective mindset. And that can only come about if opinion formers, leading practitioners, policy makers and academic leaders take 'time out' to reflect on and then attempt to modify the way they work. The three-step change model, attributed to German-American psychologist Kurt Lewin, may provide a helpful template for considering how this might be achieved. Lewin (1947) argued that change cannot be brought about by either fiat or mere argument. In his view, what is necessary is a systematic approach that takes account of the very real psychological and practical obstacles to reform. In essence, Lewin proposed that three stages – summarised as 'unfreeze, implement, refreeze' – are necessary to effect fundamental change in the mode of working of an individual, group or organisation. The three stages involve challenging existing attitudes and behaviours, implementing the necessary changes in a manner that makes sense to the stakeholders, and finally engineering a scenario that renders the changes permanent and sustainable. (This model finds echoes in the 'diagnosis, treatment, follow-up' approach to public health adopted in this book.)

A WAY FORWARD

To reposition the international public health community to meet the challenge of world health more effectively in the future, to unfreeze some of the more traditional and unfruitful patterns of thinking, to facilitate the process of making a 'diagnosis' of global health status and to adopt the appropriate and effective 'treatment' strategies, several steps are required:

1 recognise that current approaches are inadequate and that fresh ideas are urgently needed to re-energise the vision for global public health
2 identify the key principles that should underlie future strategy development
3 elaborate these principles into achievable goals or operational objectives
4 translate the goals into specific actions
5 consider how the impact of the actions may be evaluated.

The first of these five points may be taken as read (literally, in the case of those readers who have reached this point in the book); it is intrinsic to the decision to undertake the task of making a global health diagnosis. Yet even those committed to embarking on that task may encounter difficulty in sustaining their personal motivation. First, the twin challenges of scale and complexity are so enormous that many practitioners will simply become overwhelmed and seek professional rewards elsewhere. Second, the international community has created an elaborate and expensive global infrastructure, in the form of the various UN-related agencies such as the World Health Organization (WHO) and the World Bank, to tackle these problems and that may prompt the response that 'we're doing it already'. Third, the very successes of global public health – declining child mortality, increasing life expectancy, the elimination of several killer infections – breed a degree of complacency. Finally, change may be resisted because it is perceived as a destabilising and possibly high-risk distraction from entrenched routines.

For all these reasons, we need to 'unfreeze' existing modes of thinking so that the need for change is accepted. The case for change in our approach to global public health has been presented in the previous chapters. The remaining four points – elaborating principles, objectives, actions and evaluation methods – are no less challenging and are addressed in the remainder of this chapter and elsewhere in this book.

ARTICULATING THE KEY PRINCIPLES

What are the key strategic principles on which to base revitalised future public health policy making at a global level? Many candidate principles could be considered. These would have to take account of the key influences on the contemporary public health scene. Identifying these influences is a matter of subjective judgement rather than scientific analysis, although the latter will inform the former. Some frontrunners might include recognising the importance of holism in the conceptualisation of public health, the need to take account of the growing evidence base derived from research on the efficacy of public health interventions, the insights gained into human development and disease causation by viewing the human life cycle as a whole, the necessity for creating delivery vehicles for the implementation of public health interventions, the ethical imperatives of professional standard setting, transparency and accountability, and the complexity of strategy development in global public health.

The factors listed above reflect much of the content of this book. I have attempted to rearticulate them as five *key principles*.

1 Embrace a holistic view of health and disease on which to base public health responses.
2 Apply a pragmatic evidence-based approach to public health policy making and practice.
3 Adopt a lifecourse perspective on public health analysis and intervention.
4 Create efficient and transparent governance processes for public health action.
5 Strive for a comprehensive strategic overview of public health policy making and practice.

These principles, if accepted, may then be translated into more specific goals that can, in turn, be turned into action points in the context of global public health policy or strategy development.

PRINCIPLE 1: EMBRACE A HOLISTIC VIEW OF HEALTH AND DISEASE ON WHICH TO BASE PUBLIC HEALTH RESPONSES

The first priority is to try to secure international agreement on what is meant by the terms health and public health. In the Introduction, some of the difficulties involved in doing this were outlined. Agreeing on the meaning and implications of these concepts involves more than merely defining them as philosophical abstractions; it is also about understanding what we are trying to achieve – and how it will be achieved – in the context of global public health.

A useful starting point for any discussion of public health principles is the WHO (1974) definition of health: 'a state of complete physical, mental and social wellbeing and not merely the absence of disease or infirmity'.

Whatever criticisms the WHO definition may have attracted, its twin key messages have been largely accepted: that health is multifaceted, going well beyond purely biological descriptors, and that health has positive as well as negative dimensions. The holistic (all-encompassing) approach to health epitomised by this definition stresses a broad view of health along with one that recognises the mutual interdependence of its various dimensions. The holistic approach is often juxtaposed against the narrow biomedical model of health allegedly favoured by the medical profession. This canard should be laid to rest as it sets up a false dichotomy. Holism seeks to integrate different perspectives in health in a way that adds up to a coherent whole. There need be no contradiction between holistic and biomedical models of health. Both are valid in their own terms, as are traditional views of public health that are often accused by advocates of holism of being excessively preoccupied with disease prevention rather than health improvement.

All these perspectives are capable of being integrated into a singe, larger vision of public health. What is that vision? Here are a few of its core concepts. Health is indivisible – its physical, mental and social components are inextricably interlinked and Cartesian mind–body dualism has been consigned to history. Health is also relative, both within and between individuals, communities, nations and regions, and a state of absolute health is illusory. Health is a positive attribute and not merely the absence of disease or disability. Health improvement requires an understanding of the 'natural history of health' or salutogenesis (Antonovsky 1979) as a corollary to the 'natural history of disease' or pathogenesis.

If health comprises physical, psychological and social dimensions, it follows that public health practitioners should engage with all three. They should strive to develop salutogenic (health-promoting) as well as anti-pathogenic (disease-preventing) solutions to public health challenges; promote the creation of safe, nurturing and sustainable environments as well as behavioural or lifestyle changes; and recognise and exploit the untapped potential of healthcare, including clinical medicine, for further improvements to population health. They should do all of this through their health improvement and health protection roles, supplemented by their growing responsibilities to reduce health inequalities and preserve the natural environment.

All these ideas may be difficult to integrate into a single statement of principle that will secure widespread agreement from the key stakeholders. Nevertheless, the articulation and endorsement of a statement that describes health holistically are crucial for global public health strategy development as everything else is firmly predicated on it.

PRINCIPLE 2: APPLY A PRAGMATIC EVIDENCE-BASED APPROACH TO PUBLIC HEALTH POLICY MAKING AND PRACTICE

In keeping with the prevailing ethos of 'evidence-based practice' that is now dominating the world of clinical medicine, public health professionals are coming under increasing pressure to justify their actions in terms of the published research evidence. The intention is laudable – to ensure that scarce resources are invested in measures that are likely to yield real benefits to the population. Yet there is a widespread misconception, even among many seasoned professionals, about the nature of 'evidence-based' public health practice. As with evidence-based clinical practice, the public health practitioner is not required to suspend professional judgement and slavishly adopt rigidly prescribed guidelines that have been derived from systematic literature reviews. So what exactly is the 'evidence-based' approach?

Sackett and Straus (1998) defined evidence-based medicine (EBM) as 'the integration of best research evidence with clinical expertise and patient values'. Much initial opposition to EBM arose from a fear of 'recipe book medicine' in which hard-won clinical skills, learned through a long-established professional training and apprenticeship system, would be marginalised. Sackett and his colleagues responded that their intention was not to undermine clinical judgement but quite the opposite: to refine it through the application, where appropriate, of high-quality evaluational research findings, mostly generated by clinical trials, systematic reviews and related methods. They argued that a better understanding of the practical implications of the research evidence would bolster, not undermine, clinical judgement. Moreover, they introduced a third and frequently forgotten component to EBM – the perspective of the patient. This led Sackett and his colleagues to formulate a triangulation model represented as a Venn diagram in which the three discrete dimensions overlap to create a shared space in which EBM is practised. The model predicts that the differing perspectives of the doctor and the patient, supplemented by the findings of high-quality research, combine synergistically to enhance clinical skill and improve clinical outcomes. This was subsequently elaborated by others (including Spring and Hitchcock 2009) to represent evidence-based practice in psychology and other fields (Figure 8.1).

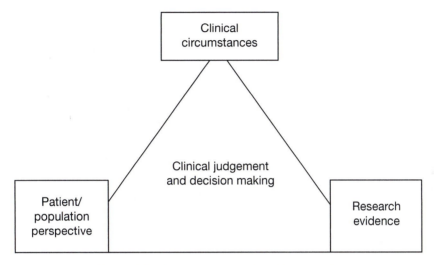

Figure 8.1 The evidence-based practice triangle.

How might these ideas about clinical and behavioural decision making be transferred to the world of public health?

Practising evidence-based public health

Evidence-based public health policy making and practice is a process of triangulation that comprises three elements: an assessment of the scientific evidence, the specific nature and circumstances of the problem, and the perspective of the target population (the 'patient'). These have to be integrated into a decision-making process that draws on all three and may be characterised as practitioner expertise.

Assessing the evidence

The rapid rise in the number of public health research papers in recent decades is a welcome trend. An expanding evidence base should better inform decision making about which measures and programmes should be deployed to address public health problems. On the other hand, the increasing volume of data has become so overwhelming that practitioners struggle to absorb it and draw appropriate lessons for practice. That was the impetus for the development of the related methods of critical appraisal and systematic reviews, whereby specialist researchers distil large tracts of published literature down to their essential, bottom-line messages for practitioners.

Critical appraisal is the process of systematically assessing research reports to judge their trustworthiness, value and relevance in a particular context. Critical appraisal (Greenhalgh 1997) has helped in the categorisation of research findings into a so-called hierarchy of evidence. This ranges from expert opinion or received wisdom (the lowest level of evidence) to systematic reviews and meta-analyses (the highest level of evidence). Occupying an intermediate position in this evidence hierarchy are randomised controlled trials (RCTs). The interpretation and summarising of research evidence in this way have become increasingly standardised and disseminated through the work of specialised researchers associated with organisations such as the Cochrane Collaboration.

Professional judgement

Research evidence should never be viewed in splendid isolation from the problems it is employed to solve. Professionals must decide, on a case-by-case basis, what action to take based upon their understanding of the nature, robustness and applicability of the evidence. The defining characteristic of any professional is the capacity to exert independent judgement that derives from the acquisition of skills during a recognised, standardised and documented training process.

Professional judgement comes into its own when research evidence is absent, inadequate, ambiguous or contentious. Not all preventive measures need to be based on RCTs and indeed, RCTs and such studies may not have been performed for good reasons. RCTs are only necessary when there is *equipoise* (uncertainty about the likely value of one course of action compared to another) between two (or more) alternatives. And not all research findings should be automatically translated into action without taking account of the wider social, political and economic context.

Involving the public

There is a tendency in some official circles to believe that large sections of the general public, particularly in disadvantaged communities, are uninformed about public health matters. That view has led to an excessive reliance on educational campaigns to banish this presumed ignorance. A more nuanced approach is to recognise the need for public engagement (or even empowerment) to facilitate public health practice.

The UK NHS, for example, has committed itself to public involvement in a way that goes beyond either educating or simply consulting people either individually or in groups. Here is a typical statement from the English Department of Health (2004).

> Effective patient and public involvement is fundamental to an NHS based on choice, responsiveness and equity. Delivering and designing health services around the needs of patients is key to the modernisation of the NHS and is integral to improving patients' experiences of health services ... The involvement of patients and the public in health decision-making is now a central theme of national and local policy in the NHS. Involvement illuminates the patient experience and helps to shape a health service that is truly responsive to individual and community needs.

Ensuring public involvement in professional or organisational decision making is far from straightforward. 'People power' is too often synonymous with the hijacking of a cause by special interest groups who may hold eccentric, prejudiced or ill-informed views about the issue in question. On occasions, positions expressed by such groups may be judged irrelevant, inappropriate or even harmful. As with the other two elements of evidence-based public health practice, public opinion should not be elevated to a uniquely unassailable status when a professional judgement is made.

All three components of an evidence-based approach – assessing the evidence, professional judgement and involving the public – are equally important in most forms of public health practice. All should be considered when planning a public health intervention or policy though it may not always prove possible to activate all of them in equal measure. Arguably, identifying the evidence base on which to base decisions about interventions is the easiest of the three from a technical point of view. Unfortunately much of the necessary evidence is simply non-existent. Identifying the gaps in evidence and allocating resources to fill them through good-quality research is an essential element in the pursuit of an evidence-based public health strategy. This is a complex subject to which we will return at various points, particularly in Chapter 12.

PRINCIPLE 3: ADOPT A LIFECOURSE PERSPECTIVE ON PUBLIC HEALTH ANALYSIS AND INTERVENTION

As described in Chapter 4, the traditional age-specific approach to the epidemiological study of human health and its determinants is steadily giving way to a lifecourse one involving the testing of biological programming and other causal hypotheses. Physical, mental and social dimensions of health are influenced by gene–environment interactions from (and sometimes before) the moment of conception. Events in early childhood can make an impact throughout the rest of life. The old saying that 'the child is father to the man' appears to be receiving increasing support from epidemiologists in the 21st century.

If the whole of the lifecourse is worth examining for the purposes of aetiological research, does not logic dictate that we do the same in the interests of population health improvement? The answer must be affirmative but caution is required. Because early influences on the developing fetus, infant and child are implicated in the risk of later disease, it does not follow that early intervention will necessarily yield the expected health benefits. A casual factor must be amenable to modification or removal, and that may not always achieve the desired result. At a theoretical level, improving maternal nutrition, for example, should improve health outcomes for children and adults but that is merely a hypothesis, albeit a plausible one, that requires formal testing by experimental methods. Only then can we feel confident, based on empirical research, that early intervention is justified. Fortunately, evidence is steadily accumulating that early intervention will indeed reap health benefits in later life. Examples of such interventions include genetic counselling, antenatal and neonatal screening for congenital anomalies, sensory screening in young children, vitamin supplementation, the encouragement of breastfeeding, immunisations, support for single parents, preschool enrichment programmes and the provision of high-quality healthcare for mothers and children.

The practical implications of the wholehearted adoption of a lifecourse approach to public health are startling and often run counter to historical precedent. We need to take radical action to try to:

➤ break down the barriers between disciplines and agencies that have responsibilities for different age groups
➤ start intervening from the very start of the life and sustain unremitting effort right through to the end
➤ include long-term outcomes, including intergenerational ones, into the operational objectives of public health plans and strategies
➤ reassess past and current strategic and local priorities to reflect the need for early intervention
➤ build capacity by equipping practitioners with the skills that will enable them to intervene effectively right across the lifecourse.

Above all, we need to follow the logic of Heckman (2008) and reallocate resources, financial and otherwise, from adults and older people to earlier in the life cycle. This policy will provoke considerable opposition and has to be advocated in a professionally responsible and politically acceptable manner, particularly in times of economic austerity (Figure 8.2).

PRINCIPLE 4: CREATE EFFICIENT AND TRANSPARENT GOVERNANCE PROCESSES FOR PUBLIC HEALTH ACTION
Two kinds of public health failure
Because public health deals in long time scales and operates across many sectors of government, success can be elusive or at least difficult to measure. A

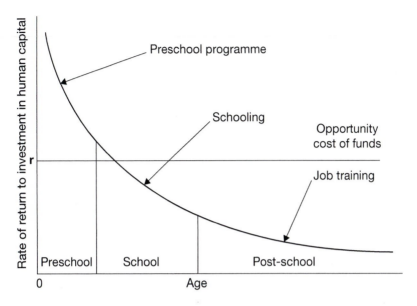

Figure 8.2 Why children are a good investment. Source: Heckman (2008).

great danger lurks here. There is a tendency on the part of some practitioners to adopt a fatalistic attitude that verges on passivity. Articulating grand visions and ambitious goals without indicating how and when they will be achieved, or how progress will be monitored, is tantamount to self-indulgence. It is also unethical. Public health should not merely be aspirational; to be effective, it must be practical and outcome oriented. Well-intentioned strategies, policies, plans and blueprints that have never been implemented abound. Many have been consigned to libraries or office shelves, condemned to gather dust for eternity.

At the opposite extreme are public health measures that are implemented with a vigour (or even zealotry) that is inappropriate or harmful. Interventions that are unsupported by convincing research evidence may be imposed on an unsuspecting public. Programmes that compromise ethical guidelines, or impinge on human rights such as individual liberty or privacy, may be rolled out without adequate prior consultation or discussion. Priorities may be set that favour some population subgroups at the expense of others or that divert scarce resources away from existing and highly valued services.

The need for good public health governance
The public health community comprises, generally speaking, public servants who receive funds from governments, charities, commercial organisations or other bodies for the purpose of improving the health of the populations for which they are responsible. All involved in public health policy making, prac-

tice and administration have an obligation to contribute to the strengthening of the credibility of public health. Creating governance procedures for ensuring accountability and transparency will nurture public confidence in public health professionals and agencies. That involves striving for a consensus around the nature of ethical public health policy and practice within the context of robust quality assurance and legal frameworks. Other key components of good governance include mechanisms for assessing the financial costs and benefits of potential interventions, for planning, delivering and monitoring intersectoral public health, and for the boosting of public health capacity through education, training and career development.

Many of these issues will be explored further in later chapters.

PRINCIPLE 5: STRIVE FOR A COMPREHENSIVE STRATEGIC APPROACH TO PUBLIC HEALTH POLICY MAKING AND PRACTICE
Process of public health policy development
A policy or strategy can be simply defined (Schopper *et al* 2006) as: 'a written document that provides the basis for action to be taken jointly by the government and its non-governmental partners'.

The WHO highlights the importance and pitfalls of national and international policy development, emphasising the need for leadership, advocacy, stakeholder involvement and an intersectoral approach. Equally vital are two further steps – implementation and evaluation (*see* Chapter 6). Note that these steps are wholly consistent with the public health approach ('diagnosis' – 'treatment' – 'follow-up') described earlier. Taken together, all these ingredients comprise the related processes of public health policy making, planning and strategy development.

Need for an integrated approach to public health policy making
Strategic policy making is cross-cutting. That is extremely challenging because governments are always organised in vertical departments. This results in a 'silo mentality' that is inefficient and obstructs progress. Numerous key national government agencies have remits and responsibilities that should be considered in public health policy making. They include healthcare, social services, education, justice, housing, transport, environment and industry. Adopting an integrated approach should help to promote coherence, enhance synergies across sectors, identify gaps, inconsistencies and duplication, allocate sufficient resources and increase visibility.

National policy making is fraught with theoretical and practical difficulties. Few countries have such comprehensive policies for public health as a whole. Most policy statements focus only on one specific topic and emanate from a single sector, thereby rendering interagency collaboration less likely.

And supranational policy or strategy development merely adds further to the already challenging nature of the task due to the multiplicity of sectors, agencies and individuals who have to be involved in the scaling up from national to international action.

Strategic policy development may be horizontal or vertical. The former strives to produce an integrated strategy that spans agencies, departments and disciplines with the aim of influencing multiple outcomes, while the latter is highly focused on measures aimed at one disorder or group of related disorders. These are not mutually exclusive positions. The decision to adopt a cross-cutting intersectoral approach, often embracing fields as diverse as health, education, housing, transport, justice and the environment, does not preclude the parallel development of more narrowly based policies designed to address specific problems. On the contrary, such a dual-track approach may be regarded as complementary, synergistic and mutually reinforcing.

If policies and strategies are to have any credibility, they must be carried through to effective implementation. That is where serious obstacles often arise. Translating high-level goals and objectives into specific actions is a skilled, time-consuming and sometimes frustrating process. The creation of efficient delivery or implementation vehicles, combined with robust monitoring or evaluation mechanisms, has to be an integral part of planning. And the system must be sufficiently flexible to respond rapidly and appropriately to unexpected or uncomfortable insights produced in the course of evaluation.

These ideas are discussed in greater detail in the next chapter.

REFERENCES

Antonovsky A. *Health, Stress and Coping.* San Francisco: Jossey-Bass; 1979.

Department of Health. *Patient and public involvement in health: the evidence for policy implementation.* 2004.

Greenhalgh T. Getting your bearings (deciding what the paper is about). *BMJ.* 1997; 315: 243–6.

Heckman JJ. Schools, skills and synapses. *Economic Inquiry.* 2008; 46(3): 289–324.

Lewin K. Frontiers of group dynamics. *Human Relations.* 1947; 1: 5–41.

Sackett DL, Straus SE. Finding and applying evidence during clinical rounds: the 'evidence cart'. *JAMA.* 1998; 280(15): 1336–8.

Schopper D, Lormand J-D, Waxweiler R, editors. *Developing Policies to Prevent Injuries and Violence: guidelines for policy-makers and planners.* Geneva: World Health Organization; 2006.

Spring B, Hitchcock K. Evidence-based practice in psychology. In: Weiner IB, Craighead WE, editors. *Corsini's Encyclopedia of Psychology.* 4th ed. New York: Wiley; 2009.

World Health Organization. Constitution of the World Health Organization. *Chron World Health Organ.* 1974; 1: 29–43.

CHAPTER 9

From principles to action

The whole point of a strategy is to work out where we want to go in relation to where we are now, and to indicate how we are going to get there. The destination – described by the mission statement or vision – is the foundation on which the bulk of the strategy (comprising principles, goals and interventions) has to be constructed. Whether or not the vision seems realistic and achievable within the constraints of available resources or time is, in a sense, beside the point; it sets the course for the journey. And the successful completion of the process involves performing tasks (action points) that are guided by signposts (goals) that point us in the right direction (principles) that will lead to the ultimate destination (vision).

FROM PRINCIPLES TO GOALS

Principles encompass the underlying values that underpin all the activities necessary to fulfil the mission statement or vision. The principles, in themselves, are non-prescriptive (*see* Chapter 8). They derive from multiple origins, including an awareness of the accumulating research evidence on a range of public health issues, and a commitment to core ethical and professional values. To formulate the precise nature, endpoint and purpose of an action point, each principle requires elaboration into more specific *goals* or objectives. What follows below is a list of 20 goals, four for each of the five principles, based on the rationale presented in the preceding chapter. Thereafter, each of the 20 goals is subdivided into three related action points.

The final structure of the proposed global public health strategy comprises a vision or mission statement (based on a set of shared values), five principles, 20 goals and 60 action points (*see* Appendix).

PRINCIPLE 1: EMBRACE A HOLISTIC APPROACH TO HEALTH AND DISEASE ON WHICH TO BASE PUBLIC HEALTH RESPONSES

Few will argue with the premise that a holistic approach is necessary for public health action. How can we translate this principle into a series of strategic purposes, goals or endpoints to which interventions should be aiming? To do this, we need to analyse the components of holism, in this context of public health, in more detail.

As discussed in the previous chapter, the holistic approach to health (and thus public health) is an inclusive, all-embracing one. This implies that all three of its dimensions – physical, mental and social – should be recognised, analysed and acted upon by policy makers and practitioners; that salutogenic (health-promoting) interventions should be included in public health strategy development along with anti-pathogenic (disease prevention) ones; that attempts to bring about lifestyle or behaviour change should be complemented by measures to create safe, health-nurturing and sustainable environments; and that the potentially important contribution of individualistic healthcare to public health should be acknowledged.

The phrase 'preventive medicine' has an old-fashioned ring. It has been criticised, perhaps unfairly, for being rooted in individualistic healthcare, for its lack of conceptual clarity, for giving undue prominence to relative risk in individuals at the expense of population-attributable risk, for underestimating the interconnected nature of risk factors, and for virtually ignoring equity in health (Starfield *et al* 2008). All these deficiencies should be remediable, in the context of a holistic public health movement, without losing the valuable contribution that preventive medicine, as a concept, can make.

Exhorting people to adopt healthier lifestyles as the mainstay of health improvement efforts is a largely discredited approach, as is expecting greater investment in the healthcare sector to deliver health gains on the necessary scale. Research suggests that, while both life circumstances and lifestyles are important determinants of health, neither is easy to change through targeted individualistic approaches. Moreover, disease-specific strategies, while important and sometimes effective, are an inadequate means of achieving significant overall population health improvements. The alternative (or at least complementary) option is to adopt broader strategies designed to direct attention on more than one disorder at a time, to refocus attention 'upstream' and create an environment that nurtures good health through salutogenesis as well as preventing poor health by protecting against pathogenesis.

Salutogenesis can operate at both individual and population levels. The availability of nutritious food from early pregnancy into old age, the promotion of adequate exercise in childhood, the provision of high-quality housing, education and other public services in disadvantaged communities, the encouragement of strong social networks, the creation of attractive leisure and recreational facilities, and the nurturing of resilient neighbourhoods are all examples of a broad-based (horizontal), upstream, salutogenic approach targeted at the whole population.

Refocusing public health attention on the environment is especially difficult in a political and professional climate that views health promotion almost
entirely through the lens of lifestyle change. Although the severe limitations of
an exclusively individualist and behavioural approach to health improvement
are well recognised, diverting public health resources towards the environmental end of the spectrum is notoriously difficult. In many countries, the problem
is compounded by history: the traditional conceptualisation of 'environmental
health', even when rebranded within 'health protection', is somewhat narrow
as it tends to address a predominantly legislative and regulatory enforcement
agenda that seldom strays outside its familiar concerns with atmospheric pollution, chemical toxicity and infectious disease control. Opportunities abound
to extend greatly the environmental approach to health improvement through
working with agencies and professionals responsible for transport, housing,
education, communities, leisure, sport and business. All these sectors can play
a role in creating an environment that is simultaneously less hazardous to
human communities and more nurturing of their health and wellbeing.

Public health commentators have often been rather dismissive of the role of
healthcare in population health improvement. While historically understand-
able, that is no longer a tenable position. First, many public health programmes
depend on a collaboration between epidemiologists, healthcare administrators,
public health personnel and clinicians for the effective and efficient planning,
implementation and evaluation of interventions. Large-scale immunisation campaigns and early disease detection through screening programmes are two obvious examples. Second, high-quality healthcare can, in itself, produce measurable
improvements in population health and quality of life, including improving case
fatality rates through the development of more effective treatments and well-co-
ordinated teamwork whether in acute hospital or community settings. Countless millions of patients have benefited from the improving prognoses of cancer,
severe trauma and cardiovascular disease – just three notable examples of the
way in which better clinical care can improve population health. In primary care,
the identification and treatment of chronic disease risk factors in adults through
either mass or opportunistic screening have also yielded substantial benefits to
population health. The bottom-line conclusion is this: healthcare should now be
regarded as a valuable health improvement tool and an integral component of
broad-based, holistic public health.

We can express these general ideas about holism in public health in a more
focused way as a list of four goals and 12 related action points (three for each goal).

Principle 1: holism
Four goals
➤ Ensure that physical, mental and social health dimensions are all
integrated into public health strategies.

➤ Seek salutogenic as well as anti-pathogenic solutions to public health challenges.
➤ Promote the creation of safe, nurturing and sustainable environments as well as behavioural/lifestyle changes.
➤ Recognise and exploit the untapped potential of healthcare for the improvement of population health through primary, secondary and tertiary prevention.

Twelve action points

1 Integrate all three dimensions of health – physical, mental and social – into all public health policy and practice, whether in the fields of health protection, health improvement or healthcare management.
2 In assessing population health, include indicators of all three dimensions of health – physical, mental and social – in both the positive sense (well-being) and negative sense (absence of disease or disability).
3 In mounting public health responses to population health challenges, seek to influence all three dimensions of health – physical, mental and social – in an integrated fashion.
4 Nurture a salutogenic (health-promoting) as well as a pathogenic (disease causation) perspective on all aspects of public health policy and practice.
5 In addition to developing and implementing disease prevention measures, identify and promote resilience and related characteristics of individuals, families, communities and populations that promote and improve positive health.
6 Adopt cross-cutting 'horizontal' approaches (notably poverty reduction), that seek to influence multiple health outcomes, to public health policy and practice, as well as adopting 'vertical' or single outcome approaches.
7 Recognise that the environment factors – physical, emotional and social – are at least as important as behaviour and healthcare in preventing disease and improving health.
8 Shift the dominant focus of health improvement activity away from behavioural or lifestyle change and individualistic healthcare towards environmental modification.
9 Expand the remit of health protection and environmental health beyond traditional concerns of pollution and infection to include the creation of safe, nurturing (salutogenic) and sustainable environments.
10 Discard divisive and unhelpful theoretical and practical distinctions between the work of public health and healthcare practitioners and policy makers.
11 Recognise the contribution of healthcare interventions and systems to the achievement of public health objectives in the training and organisation of practitioners in both fields.

12 Integrate health improvement, health protection and healthcare practitioners and systems into public health policy making and practice.

PRINCIPLE 2: APPLY A PRAGMATIC EVIDENCE-BASED APPROACH TO PUBLIC HEALTH POLICY MAKING AND PRACTICE

The critical appraisal of scientific evidence is a skilled, time-consuming and prolonged process that often appears to clash with the time scales and pressures of daily life in government departments. Professional advisors are, in theory, well placed to distil the evidence base (at least from sources of secondary data such as the Cochrane Collaboration) for policy makers but in practice often struggle to accomplish what may seem a daunting and never-ending task. The result is the existence of a widely acknowledged implementation gap between knowledge and practice.

Epidemiology is central to the practice of evidence-based public health. Among its various roles in strategic planning, three are especially noteworthy: assessing need through the analysis of routine vital statistical data, supplemented by other sources, to assess the health status of a population, and to undertake aetiological and evaluational research to enable interventions to be developed and implemented more effectively.

An important part of needs assessment is deciding where to direct scarce resources. Epidemiologists have long argued that a preventive approach that 'targets the tail' by focusing only on high-risk groups is likely to prove less effective than one that seeks to 'shift the population distribution to the left' (Rose 1985). The arguments in favour of 'curve shifting', whereby risk is reduced in the whole population, have been well rehearsed in relation to biological variables such as blood pressure and cholesterol. Less recognition is accorded to their validity in the spheres of behaviour and environment. A notable topical example that straddles both is cigarette smoking. The UK and several other jurisdictions have taken a great step forward in creating a healthier environment for all – smokers and non-smokers – by the ban on smoking in enclosed public spaces. The ban on indoor smoking has had a positive effect on both smoking prevalence and health outcomes, far exceeding the disappointing results achieved by conventional health education campaigns directed exclusively at smokers. A second example is injury prevention. The implementation of traffic-calming measures in built-up urban areas, by reducing the average speed of all traffic rather than identifying and eliminating the minority of 'high speeders', has been instrumental in achieving substantial reductions in pedestrian injury rates in many countries.

But the role of epidemiology goes much wider than the identification of priorities for the targeting of resources. Because the 'patient' is the population, a whole-population or epidemiological approach is the most rational way to assess need, select appropriate interventions and evaluate progress. This notion may appear self-evident to the public health community but cannot be assumed to command widespread acceptance among the ranks of healthcare practitioners and health policy makers in general.

Assessing need depends on the collection, analysis and interpretation of good-quality data. Some countries, like the UK, are fortunate in having an outstanding series of routine mortality and healthcare databases. Even there, serious gaps in information remain on the incidence and prevalence of many important conditions, the frequency of risk factor exposure, the prevalence and nature of disability, long-term sequelae of disease, injury and healthcare, and the quality of life of sufferers and survivors of illness and injury.

Selecting and *planning appropriate interventions* requires the deployment of highly sophisticated critical appraisal skills to assess the quality of evidence relating to the proposed interventions. However, such skills are in short supply in public health policy-making circles. The increasing involvement of 'arm's length' expert advisory bodies such as the Cochrane Collaboration and the UK National Institute for Health and Clinical Excellence (NICE) in the assessment of preventive interventions should help to remedy this shortcoming though the time scale is liable to be protracted.

Evaluating progress following the implementation of an intervention is perhaps an even more problematic area than the implementation itself. Conceptual confusion abounds with terms such as efficacy and effectiveness, research and audit, monitoring and surveillance being used interchangeably and at times inappropriately. Above all, separating out the effects of the intervention being evaluated from the effects of any underlying secular trends or other (confounding) factors unrelated to the intervention may present almost insoluble methodological obstacles.

The logic of 'evidence-based medicine' dictates that it should not be confined to clinical practice but should extend to public health in general and health improvement measures (including policy making) in particular. As in clinical practice, however, experienced professional judgement, allied with an awareness of public perceptions, is often required in the absence of high-quality scientific data. Nevertheless, the volume of robust research evidence relating to the efficacy of specific public health interventions is rapidly growing. Unfortunately, the application of such knowledge may be hampered by political timidity rather than scientific uncertainty. Two examples from the UK (that incidentally also meet the 'environmental' principle outlined earlier) are fluoridation of the water supply for the prevention of dental caries, and folate fortification of flour to reduce the risk of neural tube defects in high-risk areas. In both cases, hostile public opinion was perceived by politicians to limit options for decisive action. When public perception, the third component of the evidence-based triangle, automatically over-rides the other two (research evidence and professional judgement), effective public health is seriously undermined.

A common scenario faced by public health practitioners and policy makers is the absence of a strong evidence base on which to draw in designing specific community-based interventions rather than in articulating broad strategic aspirations. There may be good evidence that reducing the exposure of children to second-hand tobacco smoke, for example, is beneficial to respiratory health but no research-based guidance as to how this might be achieved in practice. Inadequate research planning hinders the plugging of gaps in knowledge about the efficacy of specific interventions. Practitioners should encourage funding bodies, including government-supported research councils, to commission research designed to inform detailed, pragmatic public health decision making.

Here is a translation of these reflections on evidence-based public health into four goals and 12 related action points.

Principle 2: evidence-based approach
Four goals

➤ Use epidemiology to convert data into information, knowledge and understanding as well as to assess, monitor and address need.
➤ Appraise evidence critically and systematically and disseminate the insights to practitioners and policy makers.
➤ Take account of public perceptions without succumbing to popular prejudice.
➤ Generate new knowledge about health and disease by supporting goal-oriented public health research.

Twelve action points

1 Expand the use of epidemiological approaches to assess need, select appropriate interventions and evaluate progress.
2 Build capacity in epidemiology to ensure that epidemiological and related data are appropriately analysed, interpreted and acted upon.
3 Advocate greater use of 'shifting the distribution curve to the left' rather than 'targeting the tail' in the development of public health strategy development.
4 Secure strong commitment from the global public health community to an evidence-based approach to policy and practice.
5 Subject all existing and proposed public health policies, strategies, plans, programmes and other interventions to an 'evidence-based audit'.
6 Boost capacity in the critical appraisal of the research literature to facilitate the transfer of knowledge from researchers to practitioners.
7 Involve the general public, as key stakeholders, in the planning, delivery and evaluation or monitoring of all public health interventions.

8   Consult sensitively with vulnerable groups such as children, the elderly and other minorities, in the planning, delivery and evaluation or monitoring of all public health interventions.

9   Respond to reasonable public concerns about a public health intervention without jeopardising its beneficial impact.

10 Identify major gaps in knowledge about the epidemiology, causes, treatment and prevention of diseases, as well as about health improvement, and commission appropriate goal-oriented research to fill them.

11 Develop mechanisms for knowledge transfer between public health researchers and practitioners via translational research and other forms of research dissemination.

12 Build public health research capacity through resource allocation, training and career development.

PRINCIPLE 3: ADOPT A LIFECOURSE APPROACH TO PUBLIC HEALTH ANALYSIS AND INTERVENTION

While chronic disease in adults poses a major public health challenge in all countries, focusing preventive attention on this age group will not, in itself, produce sufficient health gain because the roots of much adult ill health lie in early life. A life cycle approach is necessary whereby health improvement efforts are directed at the embryo, fetus, neonate, infant, child and adolescent as well as the middle-aged and older population groups. The work of Barker and Osmond (1986), Felitti *et al* (1998) and others has demonstrated the existence of critical developmental periods in early life (pregnancy and early childhood) during which the human organism is programmed on a trajectory of either good or poor health, physical, emotional or social. Although this trajectory may be strongly influenced by subsequent events, early life exposures and experience play a major role in influencing later health and in producing intergenerational effects. Moreover, it appears that the prospects for achieving changes in biology, life circumstances, behaviour and access to services diminish with advancing age. The earlier the intervention, the more likely it is to be effective in improving health throughout the lifecourse. Investing in parents, babies and small children will reap the greatest rewards, and the earlier the investment, the greater the return (Heckman 2008).

Early intervention should not, however, occur at the expense of later intervention, whether preventive or therapeutic. There is no point in launching children onto a path of good health in infancy and early childhood if they are liable to stumble when they reach adulthood or old age. Early intervention is thus a necessary but insufficient strategy for improving population health. In an ideal world, resources should be targeted early in the lifecourse without being withdrawn from later age groups but that may prove a vain hope in circumstances of economic scarcity.

Adopting a lifecourse approach to population health improvement is especially crucial in attempting to narrow persistent health inequalities between social, gender, ethnic and other groups. It appears to offer a possible solution to this ubiquitous policy conundrum. Poverty and socioeconomic disadvantage exert a profound impact on the developing embryo, fetus, infant and young child. That impact is manifested throughout the rest of life. If we can intervene effectively to minimise the effects of inequality at an early age, all age groups will ultimately benefit.

There are links between the manifestations and causes of health inequality and these are more often than not traceable to a single common denominator – poverty. Nevertheless, there are other potential determining factors – cultural, environmental and even (as in the case of some gender-related differences) biological. A somewhat neglected aspect of health inequality is its geographical distribution, both within and between countries. Given the extreme concentration of social deprivation – and the consequent deleterious effects on health – in specific localities, regional, nationwide or international health improvement policies may underestimate the geographical dimensions of health inequalities and thereby dilute the impact of interventions.

Health policy makers tend to adopt an assumption that geographical inequalities in health can be adequately addressed by focusing on social factors. That may be misguided: geography may influence health for many reasons – topographical, climatic and environmental – other than purely socioeconomic ones. Another social driver of geographical inequality in health is varying access to healthcare and health-promoting resources. Poorer communities cannot always easily access these facilities. Inaccessibility may be due to lack of a critical mass of skilled and committed personnel in such neighbourhoods, or because of the anomalous administrative (and hence financial) separation of areas of relative prosperity (especially the suburban hinterlands of many large cities) from the communities in greatest need, despite their geographical and functional interdependence.

What are we trying to achieve by adopting a lifecourse approach? Here are four goals and 12 related action points that flow from this principle.

Principle 3: lifecourse perspective
Four goals
➤ Start early in the human life cycle, from preconception and intergenerationally where possible.
➤ Sustain effort throughout the lifecourse unremittingly to the end of life.
➤ Reprioritise attention and resources from later to earlier in the lifecourse.
➤ Incorporate lifecourse approaches to all forms of health inequality (social, gender, ethnic, geographical) reduction.

Twelve action points

1   Adopt a long-term and intergenerational perspective on the assessment, intervention and monitoring of health across the lifecourse.
2   Focus specific attention on the practical and emotional needs of parents (especially mothers), children and families in the early part of the life-course.
3   Seek to minimise the occurrence, severity and impact of adverse childhood experiences – physical, emotional and social – in early life.
4   Integrate public health policies and practices aimed at specific objectives or age groups (such as health inequality reduction and chronic risk factor disease control) across the lifecourse.
5   Ensure that early interventions (in pregnancy, infancy and childhood) are reinforced by later ones to avoid attenuating long-term gains.
6   Focus attention on especially vulnerable stages of the lifecourse – especially the very early and very late stages – when the potential for effective intervention is greatest.
7   Advocate early intervention as an evidence-based public health strategy for the improvement of health and prevention of disease.
8   Undertake cost–benefit and other economic analyses of the likely financial return on investment in the early part of the lifecourse.
9   Shift health-promoting resources and capacity from later to earlier parts of the lifecourse without causing serious detriment to older age groups.
10 Identify commonalities and divergences between different forms of health inequality across the lifecourse.
11 Implement health inequality reduction strategies and interventions across the entire lifecourse.
12 Seek to minimise the impact of poverty, and other causes of health inequality, on the most vulnerable age groups, especially children and the elderly.

PRINCIPLE 4: CREATE EFFICIENT AND TRANSPARENT GOVERNANCE PROCESSES FOR PUBLIC HEALTH ACTION

A shortage of public health personnel is a universal complaint. Often, over-worked and dedicated practitioners have to work in stressful and poorly equipped (or even dangerous) conditions. And even where capacity exists, the competence with which the workforce performs its functions may be subopti-mal. As with all professions, good intentions are no substitute for good gover-nance – the processes and mechanisms by which responsibilities are allocated, expectations defined and performance verified. Most public health activities are publicly funded and that carries additional requirements for reassuring governments, funding bodies and the general public that expenditure is being incurred in the most efficient, effective and transparent manner. An important aspect of accountability is financial probity. Governance systems have multiple functions but are usually designed to answer one question above all others – is the allocated money being well spent?

Healthcare workers, particularly doctors and nurses, are bound by professional codes of conduct that reflect their role in society. Patients and their families are entitled to the protection that predetermined professional standards of behaviour and competence assure. Public health practitioners usually interact with communities rather than individuals and carry a great burden of responsibility for the health and welfare of those for whose benefit they are employed. Yet the ethical and legal frameworks within which public health personnel operate are often nebulous or absent.

The administrative mechanisms for delivering public health interventions efficiently and effectively are often deficient. Intersectoral co-operation should be the norm but conflicting interests or priorities may sabotage that ideal scenario. Exhorting organisations, departments, groups or individuals to work collaboratively together is usually doomed to failure. That is because internal rather than external demands will always take priority. Unless interagency working is written into job plans, with clearly defined lines of managerial responsibility and accountability, it is unlikely to happen.

Collaborative, intersectoral working is easy to endorse but hard to practise. A more effective approach is to recognise that function flows from structure and to create appropriate, practical means of applying that insight. Such structures need not be rigid and permanent – short-life task forces can prove highly effective – but they should exist. In parallel with an effort to develop fresh strategic thinking, governments must strive to secure renewed policy commitment to multisectoral health improvement, led at the highest level by the health minister. Securing this high-level support can be helped by demonstrating the economic advantages of effective public health, both in terms of greater organisational efficiency and in generating long-term savings for the public purse. A greater use of econometric research methods can contribute to promoting this understanding. Adequate administrative support and resources must also be provided to reinforce intersectoral collaboration. These should be made available over a prolonged period of decades rather than weeks or months.

Public health is only as effective as the capacity of its multidisciplinary workforce. Inadequate training and career structures, low levels of skill development and insufficient numbers of practitioners will all severely hamper national and international public health efforts. There is a worldwide shortage of public health capacity that can only be remedied by the introduction or expansion of educational and training programmes designed to meet the needs of modern public health.

To improve the quality of global public health, we need to create governance mechanisms through the following four goals and 12 related action points.

Principle 4: governance

Four goals

➤ Develop a consensus around the nature of ethical public health policy and practice within the context of robust quality assurance and legal frameworks.

➤ Take account of financial costs and benefits of potential interventions.

➤ Create appropriate mechanisms for planning, delivering and monitoring intersectoral public health.

➤ Boost high-quality public health capacity through standardised, affordable and practical education, training and career development.

Twelve action points

1   Subject public health practitioners to an ethical code of practice as robust as that applicable to doctors and other healthcare professionals.

2   Strive for an international consensus on the nature of the ethical and legal rights and obligations of public health practitioners.

3   Seek legal protection for public health practitioners who may encounter pressures, threats and other barriers to their pursuit of legitimate public health objectives.

4   Include health econometric approaches, especially cost–benefit analyses, into strategic public health planning.

5   Increase health economic capacity in academic and service departments of public health.

6   Resist the use of exclusively or predominantly economic arguments or data on which to base public health decision making.

7   Seek high-level policy endorsement for intersectoral, multidisciplinary working as the norm for all public health activity.

8   Incorporate intersectoral, multidisciplinary working into job descriptions and appraisal processes across the public health workforce.

9   Develop administrative delivery structures, backed by adequate resources, to plan, implement and monitor public health interventions including those requiring rapid responses to acute (including infectious, environmental or humanitarian) incidents.

10 Highlight the need for an expanded multidisciplinary workforce throughout the world to deliver improvements in global health.

11 Inspire, recruit and retain to the public health workforce through high-quality undergraduate and postgraduate training.

12 Provide appropriate, standardised, affordable and practical educational courses, training programmes and career structures for the public health workforce.

PRINCIPLE 5: STRIVE FOR A COMPREHENSIVE STRATEGIC APPROACH TO PUBLIC HEALTH POLICY MAKING AND PRACTICE

The theme of public health strategy development runs like a connecting thread throughout this book. In the author's view, this is the supreme principle of global public health. Without a strategy, it is impossible to plan effectively or to deliver and evaluate interventions in a coherent way. A strategic approach provides a coherent framework for public health action and offers all countries and communities the best chance of meeting the aspirations of their people for better health.

The components of a plan, policy or strategy have been explored in previous chapters. Readers may recall that a strategy is something of a paradox: it is simple in its intention (to chart a course from A to B) yet complex in its execution (depending both on the writing of the strategy itself and its implementation coupled with evaluation). To reiterate: the key requirements of successful strategy development are the articulation of an ultimate vision based on shared values and principles, their elaboration into a series of more focused goals or objectives, and a specification of the particular interventions or action points that will enable the goals to be met. All these elements may be wrapped up, along with plans for implementation and evaluation, into a single strategic document. The core of the strategy comprises the principles, goals and action points that flow from the overall vision or mission statement. One proposed version of these core elements of a global public health strategy is shown in the Appendix.

Strategy development relies on effective leadership, persuasive advocacy, engagement with stakeholders and co-operation across agencies. That is true whether the strategy is developed for local, national or international application. In today's globalised world, a collaborative transnational or supranational effort is necessary; purely national planning for public health will inevitably prove insufficient. A global infrastructure already exists (in the form of the WHO and other agencies such as the World Bank) for this purpose and much work of this type has been conducted or is planned. The full potential for global co-operation on public health remains unfulfilled and it is up to all countries, represented by their political leaders and officials (the so-called 'international community'), to exploit it further.

Developing a strategy is only the first step. Failure to implement it effectively negates the entire endeavour. The true test of strategy is whether or not it achieves its objectives. That can only be assessed through careful monitoring, either by means of formal evaluation or audit, or by periodically reviewing progress. Evaluation needs to be incorporated into the entire strategic process by means of a feedback loop, with the findings properly internalised and acted upon as swiftly as possible. Evaluation should not be regarded as optional but as an ethical imperative.

The strategic principle may be expressed as four goals and 12 related action points as follows.

Principle 5: strategy development

Four goals

➤ Identify, nurture and promote leadership and advocacy for public health across all professions and sectors.

➤ Forge strategic alliances with non-health sectors responsible for health-relevant policies such as those concerned with the economy, climate change and security.

➤ Work globally to achieve public health objectives internationally, nationally, regionally and locally.

➤ Incorporate evaluation – and the capacity to change – into all public health strategy making to enable the success or otherwise of interventions to be assessed.

Twelve action points

1 Provide additional training to suitably motivated and talented individuals to enable them to adopt leadership roles within multidisciplinary and multisectoral public health.

2 Allocate clearly defined leadership roles to sectors, agencies and individuals to facilitate public health policy making and practice.

3 Enhance public health advocacy in all relevant spheres of both public and private sector policy and practice.

4 Establish effective mechanisms for collaboration between health and non-health sectors in pursuit of public health objectives.

5 Secure a cross-sectoral consensus that the improvement and protection of population health is an important strategic policy objective.

6 Ensure that health is widely viewed across government departments and beyond as both an end in itself and as a necessary input to economic development, countering climate change, national security and other strategic objectives.

7 Raise awareness of the transnational nature of contemporary threats to population health and the need to mount global as well as national and local responses.

8 Building on existing organisations, strengthen the global public health infrastructure to optimise international co-operation and collaboration to address global health challenges.

9 Seek to integrate the various international statements, agreements, strategies and programmes into a single, overarching, streamlined global public health strategy.

10 Stress the ethical and practical imperative to evaluate all public health

interventions to ensure that precious public resources are invested in the most effective and efficient manner possible.

11 Enhance evaluational capacity through undergraduate, postgraduate and in-service training of students and practitioners.

12 Ensure that the necessary feedback loops are constructed to enable public health staff to respond appropriately to the results of evaluation and monitoring.

FROM GOALS TO ACTIONS: THE CORE OF A GLOBAL PUBLIC HEALTH STRATEGY

As we move down the strategic hierarchy from the vision (the ultimate destination) through the underpinning principles (the direction of travel) to the goals (the signposts), we can begin to see the practical implications of the strategy. This is the stage where abstract ideas become more concrete and translate into specific action points. The Appendix presents the core elements of a possible global public health strategy, based on the five principles, 20 goals and 60 action points listed in the previous section. Its purpose is twofold: to illustrate what the core elements of such a strategy might include, and to offer one possible version for debate. A key question in that debate is this: even if a consensus were to emerge that all 60 action points are worth implementing, are they all equally important? The answer is far from clear and is dependent on professional judgement and perspective. What is hardly in doubt is that some effort at prioritisation should be attempted. That is the subject of the next chapter.

REFERENCES

Barker DJP, Osmond C. Infant mortality, childhood nutrition and ischaemic heart disease in England and Wales. *Lancet.* 1986; **1**: 1077–81.

Felitti VJ, Anda RF, Nordenberg D, *et al.* Relationship of childhood abuse and household dysfunction to many of the leading causes of death in adults: the Adverse Childhood Experiences (ACE) Study. *Am J Prev Med.* 1998; **14**: 245–58.

Heckman JJ. Schools, skills and synapses. *Economic Inquiry.* 2008; **46**(3): 289–324.

Rose G. Sick individuals and sick populations. *Int J Epidemiol.* 1985; **14**: 32–8.

Starfield B, Hyde J, Gervas J, Heath I. The concept of prevention: a good idea gone astray? *J Epidemiol Commun Health.* 2008; **62**: 580–3.

CHAPTER 10

The top strategic priorities for global public health

PRIORITY SETTING: HOW IS IT DONE?

The term 'priority' implies both a ranking and a right to preferential attention of some kind. The underlying criteria that are used to identify priorities
are seldom stated explicitly. They may include importance (burden of disease
by severity, age, gender and risk factors), availability of interventions (research
evidence, technology), practicality (cost, feasibility) and timeliness (public and
professional opinion, politics). Priority setting is seldom an objective process
as it involves the exercise of judgement in selecting and ranking the preferred
actions. There are no 'right' or 'wrong' priorities, only those that can secure support or otherwise from stakeholders.

Because so many of the diseases, disorders and risk factors that afflict the
world's population can be traced back to a single common pathway, interventions that are designed to address that shared origin are especially important.
Such interventions are described as horizontal in nature. Examples include poverty reduction, better nutrition, parenting support and high-quality healthcare.
Based on my reading of the evidence on efficacious approaches, in the context
of the global health needs of the today's world, and using the 60-point strategy
proposed in the Appendix as a template, I have selected six horizontal global
public health priorities for immediate attention. Three are strategic in nature
and three are infrastructural. Without belittling any of the other elements of
the strategy, these six priorities seem to me to represent the most serious and
pressing challenges to the international public health community. Being horizontal rather than vertical in nature, they are designed to modify upstream,
intersectoral factors or circumstances relevant to a range of outcomes rather
than specific diseases or disorders.

Before exploring these horizontal priorities in detail, we need to recognise
past successes and the enduring relevance of vertical strategies and programmes.

VERTICAL STRATEGIES

Vertical strategies are aimed at the elimination or amelioration of specific diseases and risk factors. They are highly focused on a narrow range of activities and outcomes. Examples include the manufacture and distribution of therapeutic or preventive products or technologies such as vaccines, antimalarial bed nets and anti-tuberculosis (TB) drugs. Others seek to encourage health-promoting behaviours such as breastfeeding, hand hygiene and smoking cessation. Some particularly noteworthy examples are shown in Box 10.1. Many of them were planned and implemented by the World Health Organization (WHO) working with partner agencies and large numbers of public health practitioners throughout the world.

BOX 10.1 *Examples of vertical global health programmes*

➤ Stop TB
➤ Roll Back Malaria
➤ Global Alliance for Vaccines and Immunisation
➤ Global Fund to Fight against AIDS, TB and Malaria
➤ Malaria Vaccine Initiative
➤ International AIDS Vaccine Initiative
➤ Global Polio Eradication Campaign
➤ Global Alliance for the Elimination of Leprosy
➤ Lymphatic Filariasis Control Program
➤ Tropical Disease Research Program
➤ GOBI (growth monitoring, oral rehydration, breastfeeding, immunisation)
➤ Onchocerciasis Control Program

One such vertical programme eradicated smallpox several decades ago and another may soon overcome polio. Several others have had less dramatic results but nevertheless have achieved striking improvements in global health. They include initiatives aimed at chronic diseases, childhood mortality, communicable diseases and injury prevention.

Chronic disease prevention

In 2000, the World Health Assembly (WHA) endorsed the Global Strategy for the Prevention and Control of Non-communicable Diseases (NCDs). The Strategy has three objectives: mapping the epidemic of NCDs and their causes; reducing the main risk factors through health promotion and primary prevention approaches; and strengthening healthcare for people already afflicted with

NCDs (World Health Organization 2011). Subsequently, several related strategies have been pursued by the WHO, including the Framework Convention on Tobacco Control (*see* below) and strategies on diet, physical activity and alcohol. Recognising that strategies alone may be insufficient, the WHA instituted a five-year Action Plan in 2008 to try to bring about concrete measures. The Action Plan contained six objectives:

➤ to raise the priority accorded to non-communicable diseases in development work at global and national levels, and to integrate the prevention and control of such diseases into policies across government departments

➤ to establish and strengthen national policies and plans for the prevention and control of non-communicable diseases

➤ to promote interventions to reduce the main shared modifiable risk factors: tobacco use, unhealthy diets, physical inactivity and harmful use of alcohol

➤ to promote research for the prevention and control of non-communicable diseases

➤ to promote partnerships for the prevention and control of non-communicable diseases

➤ to monitor non-communicable diseases and their determinants and evaluate progress at the national, regional and global levels.

The WHO recommends 10 'best buys' for NCD prevention (Box 10.2). In addition to these, it has identified several additional cost-effective interventions: nicotine dependence treatment; promoting adequate breastfeeding and complementary feeding; enforcing drink-driving laws; restrictions on marketing of foods and beverages high in salt, fats and sugar, especially to children;

BOX 10.2 *Best buys for population-based NCD prevention*

➤ Protecting people from tobacco smoke and banning smoking in public places
➤ Warning about the dangers of tobacco use
➤ Enforcing bans on tobacco advertising, promotion and sponsorship
➤ Raising taxes on tobacco
➤ Restricting access to retailed alcohol
➤ Enforcing bans on alcohol advertising
➤ Raising taxes on alcohol
➤ Reduce salt intake and salt content of food
➤ Replacing trans-fat in food with polyunsaturated fat
➤ Promoting public awareness about diet and physical activity

and food taxes and subsidies to promote healthy diets. It also emphasises the importance of individual interventions delivered via healthcare systems, especially at primary care level.

Progress in implementing the Action Plan has been slow for various reasons, including the mistaken perception that NCDs are largely a problem for affluent countries, and that the modification of behavioural risk factors is primarily the responsibility of individuals rather than professionals or governments.

A particular focus of international concern has been the key role of smoking in the causation of much chronic disease. Almost 6 million people are estimated to die from tobacco use each year (World Health Organization 2011), a figure that is expected to increase relentlessly in the future unless serious action is taken. The WHO Framework Convention on Tobacco Control (2003) epitomises efforts to promulgate good practice in the pursuit of a single global public health goal – a reduction in tobacco-related harm. The Framework was adopted by the WHA with strong international support and came into force in 2005. Since then, it has been remarkably well received by member states and is considered one of the most successful international treaties in the UN's history. More than a set of guidelines, the Framework is a legally binding treaty that helps to bring about equitable global standards in health. The ground-breaking aspects of this initiative are the setting of international standards relating to the manipulation, for health protection purposes, of tobacco demand and supply. The multidisciplinary public health measures recommended by the Framework are designed to control tobacco price, advertising, packaging, sales to minors and illicit trade, to raise public awareness, disseminate effective educational and smoking cessation programmes, and to support economically viable alternatives. Signatory states are expected to provide periodic progress reports. While most have done so, it has become clear that implementation is extremely variable. Non-implementation rates are especially high in the fields of tobacco advertising and environmental protection from tobacco smoke. Despite its generally favourable reception, the WHO's Director General, Dr Margaret Chan, has pointed out that less than 10% of the world's population is fully protected by any of the tobacco demand-reduction measures contained in the Framework (World Health Organization 2011). Further sustained lobbying will be needed to persuade more governments to implement the Framework in full.

Childhood mortality reduction

Reducing child mortality is one of the Millennium Development Goals (MDGs). Much effort has been devoted to addressing childhood mortality and with good reason – there are more than 10 million deaths annually of children under the age of five years. Recognising the damaging effect of child mortality on both global health and economic development, the UNICEF-backed

Campaign for Child Survival has had some spectacular successes. By scaling up available technologies in low-income settings, it has contributed to sharply declining child mortality rates in the world's poorer regions, saving many millions of lives in its first decade. The Campaign promoted a package of interventions known as GOBI: growth monitoring of children, oral rehydration therapy for diarrhoeal diseases, breastfeeding to improve nutrition and immunity, and immunisation against six lethal diseases (TB, diphtheria, whooping cough, tetanus, polio and measles). In a parallel initiative, the UN launched its Global Strategy for Women's and Children's Health in April 2010 in response to concerns that the MDG on child mortality would fall substantially short of its target (United Nations 2010). This emphasised the need to redouble efforts to boost healthcare capacity in maternal and child health throughout the world but especially in sub-Saharan Africa.

The Bellagio Study Group on Child Survival, comprising a small number of concerned scientists from around the world, held a series of meetings in conjunction with the WHO, UNICEF and the World Bank. This culminated in a workshop, sponsored by the Rockefeller Foundation, in Bellagio, Italy, in 2003. The Group published an influential series of papers in *The Lancet* in that year that stimulated the 'child survival debate' in various fora. The authors claimed that implementing 23 proven and cost-effective interventions could prevent two-thirds of all child deaths (Bellagio Study Group on Child Survival 2003). To date, much emphasis has been placed upon nutrition, infection and neonatal health; injury prevention has scarcely featured in these discussions though it clearly deserves greater attention in view of its epidemiological contribution to childhood mortality.

Communicable disease control

Even countries that have traversed the epidemiological transition remain locked in a perpetual struggle against communicable diseases. Poorer countries suffer disproportionately from their impact, much of which is avoidable through the application of both therapeutic and preventive measures. The 'big three' infectious diseases – AIDS, TB and malaria – have rightly been the focus of much attention through the Global Fund, a multiagency initiative that secured policy support from the US government, the UN and the World Bank, among others. The Global Fund has had a chequered history with no shortage of critics, including those who argue that its establishment came at the expense of numerous other relatively neglected diseases such as onchocerciasis, schistosomiasis, injuries and mental illness. Nevertheless, the Global Fund and other initiatives, including the US President's Emergency Plan for AIDS Relief, have worked synergistically to bring the AIDS pandemic (that has claimed at least 25 million lives since 1981) under control. The Global Alliance for Vaccines and Immunisation was launched with the help of a $750 million grant from the Bill and Melinda Gates Foundation to boost immunisation rates in poorer countries. Within five years, 42 million children had been vaccinated against hepatitis B, and millions more against *Haemophilus influenzae* type B, yellow fever and other infections. The various campaigns against malaria instigated by the WHO have had mixed results, especially in Africa, but there is no denying some significant achievements. A combination of three measures (pesticide spraying, the use of antimalarial drugs and antimalarial bed nets) has protected well over half the world's population living in high-risk areas from endemic disease.

Injury and violence prevention

The epidemiological importance of injury worldwide has been well documented by the WHO in its series of reports on various aspects of the problem, particularly road traffic injuries (Peden *et al* 2004). The perception of injuries as a public health challenge is a relatively recent phenomenon and one that has been vigorously promoted by the WHO through its Violence and Injury Prevention and Disability initiatives (www.who.int/violence_injury_prevention/en/index.html).

Most injuries are unintentional and most of those are road traffic injuries (RTIs). Several interventions have been found to reduce RTI incidence, severity or risk. The most noteworthy are area-wide urban safety measures (such as better road design); the promotion of average traffic speed reduction in both residential and rural areas; the passage and enforcement of legislation on seatbelt/child restraint and drink-driving; universal bicycle/motorcycle helmet wearing; safer vehicle design; and community-based education/advocacy measures to protect pedestrians. Many of these measures have been implemented to great effect in high-income countries but low-income countries, where the need is greatest, have been unable or unwilling to do so. In March 2010, the United Nations General Assembly passed a resolution co-sponsored by 100 countries endorsing the launch of a Decade of Action (2011–2021) for Road Safety.

A formidable evidence-based armamentarium of countermeasures is available for many other injury types and will not be described in detail here. The basic approach to injury prevention is summarised by the three Es – education, enforcement and engineering (or environmental medication) – applied across the lifecourse. A strong emphasis on unintentional injury in most countries reflects its relative epidemiological importance compared to intentional injury. That may change as all forms of intentional injury – suicide, interpersonal violence and group violence – become relatively more frequent in most regions of the world.

In reviewing the research evidence on violence prevention, the WHO (2009), in collaboration with an academic team from Liverpool, identified seven strategies.

1   Developing safe, stable and nurturing relationships between children and their parents and caregivers.
2   Developing life skills in children and adolescents.
3   Reducing the availability and harmful use of alcohol.
4   Reducing access to guns, knives and pesticides.
5   Promoting gender equality to prevent violence against women.
6   Changing cultural and social norms that support violence.
7   Victim identification, care and support programmes.

Using the Social Ecological Model (see Chapter 1) as a template, McVeigh *et al* (2005) suggested that action be taken simultaneously and in a co-ordinated fashion at four levels: individual, relationship, community and societal. Here are their recommendations.

➤ *Individual level*: reduce unwanted pregnancies, increase access to prenatal/ postnatal services, implement child maltreatment programmes, offer social development training and provide academic enrichment programmes.
➤ *Relationship level:* provide home visiting services, parenting programmes, anti-bullying programmes and mentoring services.
➤ *Community level*: train professionals in the screening, detection and referral of victims of violence, change the culture of institutions (schools, care homes, etc.), provide co-ordinated community interventions, disrupt illegal weapon markets and implement alcohol/drug reduction strategies.
➤ *Societal level:* de-concentrate poverty, reduce inequality, strengthen police and judicial systems and reduce media violence.

Suicide prevention usually falls within the remit of the mental health sector in most countries, with a reliance on psychological screening and case finding designed to detect and treat depression. In 2001, the USA published a comprehensive National Strategy for Suicide Prevention that adopted a community-wide approach embracing public health as well as clinical measures. That resonates well with the WHO calls for a multisectoral approach within the broader context of injury prevention.

A systematic review of suicide prevention interventions (Guo and Harstall 2004) identified three broad approaches to suicide prevention:
➤ primary prevention (universal or selective)
➤ treatment (case identification and treatment)
➤ maintenance (long-term care and follow-up).

Another systematic review (Mann *et al* 2005) reported an analysis of research findings by suicide experts from 15 countries and concluded that only two interventions were supported by evidence: education of physicians in the recognition and treatment of depression (with an important caveat that the use of selective serotonin reuptake inhibitors in children required further study), and restriction of access to lethal means (such as firearm control and detoxification of domestic gas).

Overall, there is a paucity of high-quality evaluation studies of suicide preventive measures. Most of the interventions that have been studied adopt a clinical perspective rather than a total population one. The only interventions that have clearly been shown to be effective in reducing suicide rates in younger age groups are school-based interventions aimed at adolescents, physician education in suicide recognition and treatment, and restriction of access to lethal suicide means. In future, governments and professionals will need to undertake more long-term strategic thinking in addressing the global challenge of suicide and deliberate self-harm. That will involve adopting an explicitly public health approach spanning the entire life cycle, including the early years.

All of these and many other highly focused vertical programmes are likely to continue and evolve in the future. They will doubtless achieve more successes that should be applauded and reinforced by solid, long-term financial and political support from national governments and international agencies. To maximise their impact, they need to be facilitated by the launching of simultaneous and equally high-profile horizontal strategic interventions that are crosscutting, in disease terms, and help to nurture salutogenic (health-promoting) approaches rather than purely disease-preventing ones.

HORIZONTAL STRATEGIES

I propose three policy priorities for immediate *strategic action*:
1   work with others to eliminate absolute poverty and ameliorate relative poverty
2   focus on creating a healthy, safe and sustainable environment
3   start early in the lifecourse to prevent disease and improve health.

I propose three priorities for immediately improving the *infrastructure*:
1   adopt a horizontal strategic framework for global public health while continuing to deliver vertical interventions
2   improve routine health data completeness and quality
3   boost public health capacity in the form of infrastructure, skills and resources.

Priority 1: work with others to eliminate poverty and inequity

Of the roughly 7 billion inhabitants of the world, about a billion live in high-income (wealthy) countries, a billion live in extremely poor (low-income) countries and the remainder live in moderately poor (middle-income) countries. Several regions of the world have experienced sustained economic growth in the last few decades and that has had an ameliorating impact on poverty. But the picture is an uneven one. Most of the poorer countries have embarked on a trajectory of economic growth that is slowly but surely leading them towards a more prosperous, and healthier, era. The exceptions are a number of extremely poor countries – the so-called 'bottom billion' (Collier 2008).

Both the numbers and proportions of extreme poverty are rising in Africa but falling in Asia. Sachs (2005) claims that it should be possible to achieve two related objectives by 2025: to end extreme poverty and to ensure that all poor countries can progress up the ladder of economic development. The vehicle for achieving these ambitious aims is, asserts Sachs, a commitment by the international community to a 'global compact' between the rich and poor countries: the rich countries will need to move beyond platitudes and their currently inadequate efforts to provide the help required, while the poor countries will be expected to devote a greater share of their national resources to reducing poverty rather than to war, corruption and political infighting. Both sides of the equation must play their part. The key obligation on the part of rich countries is to make more money available, while that of the poor countries is to ensure good governance. The framework for implementing the compact should be the Millennium Development Goals.

Millennium Development Goals

In 2000, the General Assembly of the UN adopted, as an adjunct to the Millennium Declaration, eight Millennium Development Goals (MDGs). Their significance cannot be overstated as they are the most broadly supported, comprehensive and specific development goals the world has ever agreed upon. The goals (Box 10.3) relate to poverty, hunger, maternal and child mortality, disease, inadequate shelter, gender inequality, environmental degradation and economic development. While extremely ambitious, they are more than aspirational and are linked to action and measurable targets. Their political importance lies in the fact that they echo an appreciation by the international community, perhaps for the first time, of the mutual self-interest that renders poverty reduction a common goal for all humanity. A crucial message seems at last to have been internalised by the world's leading economists, development experts and some governments: health is a necessary prerequisite of prosperity and ill health is an inevitable outcome of poverty. The MDGs stress the multifaceted nature of poverty and the need to mount a comprehensive response that includes a major health component.

The MDGs are bound by time lines and prescribe, through recommendations linked to concrete numerical benchmarks, strategies to reduce extreme poverty. If these are achieved, by 2015, world poverty will be halved, millions of lives will be saved and billions of people will benefit from economic progress. That in turn would represent a major advance for global health. Progress

BOX 10.3 *The Millennium Development Goals.*

The Millennium Declaration, endorsed by 189 world leaders at the UN in September 2000, is a commitment to work together to build a safer, more prosperous and equitable world. The Declaration was translated into a roadmap setting out eight time-bound and measurable goals to be reached by 2015, known as the Millennium Development Goals (MDGs).

Goal 1 Eradicate extreme poverty and hunger
➤ Reduce by half the proportion of people whose income is less than $1 a day.
➤ Reduce by half the proportion of people who suffer from hunger.

Goal 2 Achieve universal primary education
➤ Ensure that all boys and girls complete a full course of primary schooling.

Goal 3 Promote gender equality and empower women
➤ Eliminate gender disparity in primary and secondary education preferably by 2005, and in all levels of education no later than 2015.

Goal 4 Reduce child mortality
➤ Reduce by two-thirds the mortality of children under five.

Goal 5 Improve maternal health
➤ Reduce maternal mortality by three-quarters.

Goal 6 Combat HIV/AIDS, malaria and other diseases
➤ Halt and reverse the spread of HIV/AIDS.
➤ Halt and reverse the incidence of malaria and other major diseases.

Goal 7 Ensure environmental sustainability
➤ Integrate principles of sustainable development into country policies and programmes, and reverse the loss of environmental resources.
➤ Halve the proportion of people without access to safe drinking water and basic sanitation.
➤ Improve the lives of at least 100 million slum dwellers by 2020.

Goal 8 Develop a global partnership for development
➤ Develop further an open, rule-based, predictable, non-discriminatory trading and financial system.
➤ Address special needs of the least developed countries, landlocked countries and small island developing states.

continued

> ➤ Deal with developing countries' debt.
> ➤ Develop and implement strategies for decent work for youth.
> ➤ Make available the benefits of new technologies, especially information and communications.
>
> Source: www.undp.org/mdg/basics.shtml.

so far appears to have been mixed: while some inroads have been made into poverty, many of the other targets are likely to be missed. Unsurprisingly, the countries lagging behind are concentrated in especially poor regions of the world, including sub-Saharan Africa and South Asia.

Goal 1 addresses poverty directly. Goals 2 and 3 suggest that gender equality and education (especially for girls) may offer a road out of poverty. Goals 4, 5 and 6 refer explicitly to health (child mortality, maternal health and communicable diseases). Goals 7 and 8 are concerned with the environment (including drinking water and sanitation) and need for global co-operation respectively. All eight goals clearly have major implications for global public health. Achievement of the MDGs will especially benefit women and children. More than half of all child deaths worldwide are associated with malnutrition and its consequences. Education is closely linked to health, and the empowerment of women will enhance their ability to raise healthy children, a view that has been reinforced by the UN's recently launched campaign to focus antipoverty measures on women. That, in turn, arose from a series of UN conferences on gender equality culminating in the General Assembly's establishment of UN Women in 2010. Maternal and child health are inextricably linked, and children are exceptionally vulnerable to unsafe and unhygienic environments. This illustrates the powerful connections between the various MDGs. Poverty reduction, education, gender equality, environmental improvement and public health are inextricably intertwined.

The MDGs, like all such declarations, have their detractors who claim that they lack focus, are not clearly correlated to intervention strategies and are more rhetorical than practical. Sachs (2005) identifies four specific concerns that could obstruct progress towards the MDGs unless they are effectively neutralised: debt, global trade policy, science for development and environmental stewardship. He calls for the debts of highly indebted poor countries to be annulled outright, for improved market access for poor countries through a liberalisation of international (especially agricultural) trade, for an expansion of research and technological investment to meet the challenges of poor countries, and for effective action to combat climate change.

The top priority for global development is to meet the basic needs – estimated by the World Bank at just over $1 per person per day – of the world's poorest billion people. The theoretical average shortfall per person is $0.31, or a total of $124 billion per year (at 2001 prices). Sachs points out that a transfer of 0.6% of income from rich to poor countries could wipe out this shortfall. This is almost identical to the 2002 Monterrey target of 0.7% to which donor countries have already committed themselves. Sachs proposes several immediate steps to be taken, including making an international commitment to end extreme poverty by 2025, adopting a global compact of rich and poor nations, reforming international institutions such as the International Monetary Fund, World Bank and United Nations, harnessing global science, promoting sustainable development, and encouraging all individuals on the planet to make a personal commitment to assist with the task.

Collier (2008) is equally positive about the prospects for eliminating 'the running sore' of extreme poverty that is concentrated in Africa and Central Asia (with a scattering elsewhere). Like Sachs, he believes that ending poverty is feasible and that it is a less daunting prospect than combating the 20th-century disasters of epidemic diseases, fascism and communism. Unlike Sachs, he seems more pessimistic about enforcing a 'global compact', arguing that we cannot rely on the governments of the poorest countries to act appropriately and decisively. The reasons relate to their well-documented inherent weaknesses and poverty traps. Foremost among these are poor governance and policies (particularly corruption and incompetence), conflict (in the form, mainly, of civil wars or coups), being geographically landlocked and surrounded by equally poor, hostile or otherwise unhelpful neighbours, and an excessive dependence on a dominant natural resource.

Collier proposes the application of four instruments: aid (carefully planned and responsive to need), robust security measures (including, where necessary, military intervention), binding international agreements (expressed in laws, standards and charters), and trading practices (driven by pragmatic rather than ideological motives). Aid has to be carefully targeted at the very poorest countries and integrated into postconflict management. Military intervention, he argues, is distasteful but sometimes necessary to restore and maintain peace, though that argument meets with strong resistance following the Iraq debacle. International charters can help to reduce corruption, improve governance and enhance accountability. Trade has to be reformed in a way that protects the poorest countries from competition, especially from the emerging Asian economies. All of these have to be tackled, he urges, in a co-ordinated manner across agencies and government departments, free of the conventional political prejudices of both the Left and the Right.

Extreme poverty of the kind that the 'bottom billion' suffer is not, of course, the whole story. Relative poverty and social inequality exert a corrosive effect on health and wellbeing throughout the world. The gap between rich and poor areas, in terms of both income and health, is widening in many countries, including the most affluent. A renewed effort to promote social mobility and achieve a more equitable distribution of income is necessary though not always politically popular. Economic growth, a goal advocated by all mainstream political parties in recent decades, may not be capable of solving this problem in affluent countries. That is because some of the unwanted side-effects of economic growth – unhealthy lifestyle, unsafe, polluted and 'obesogenic' environments, and the adverse effects of climate change – may nullify many of the potential health benefits that accompany affluence and contribute to widening social inequalities in health. 'Sustainable development' is one proposed answer. It adopts a long-term, intergenerational perspective that discourages material consumption, encourages a modal shift in transport, promotes equity and social justice, responds vigorously to climate change, and focuses on the creation of a healthy and safe built environment (Sustainable Development Commission 2010).

Priority 2: focus on creating a healthy, safe and sustainable environment

It is a paradox of contemporary public health that, while politicians and the media seem excessively preoccupied with behavioural approaches to health improvement, much knowledge has been accrued and protective action taken in the field of environmental health. Environmental agents – physical, chemical, biological, psychological and social – influence health in ways that are increasingly understood. Some of these act in isolation while others do so synergistically. At least 15 000 synthetic chemicals, a range of physical agents and several biological contaminants threaten human health. Atmospheric pollution, global warming and other potentially health-damaging forms of environmental disruption are engendering growing concern. Furthermore, there is growing recognition that the emotional, social and economic aspects of the environment are equally important to health and wellbeing. The net result is a mounting anxiety that environmentally induced disorders are on the increase in many parts of the world. These include asthma, cancers, injuries, birth defects and a variety of other conditions attributable to more subtle neurotoxic and developmental effects. Other environmentally induced disorders include respiratory and gastrointestinal diseases arising from pollution and inadequate sanitation respectively, and vector-related diseases such as malaria and schistosomiasis caused, in part, by poor drainage. Smith *et al* (1999) estimated that 25–33% of the global burden of diseases could be attributed to environmental risk factors (often associated with poverty) such as indoor air pollution (mainly due to indoor cooking), outdoor air pollution and unsafe water – a higher figure than that for both unsafe sex and tobacco use.

The impact of the environment on child health has been a particular focus of international policy attention in recent years. In 1996, the environment ministers of the G8 countries acknowledged the special vulnerability of children and committed their countries to action on several specific issues: lead poisoning, contaminated drinking water, endocrine-disrupting chemicals, environmental tobacco smoke and poor air quality. Furthermore, they asserted that preventing exposure was the most effective way of protecting children's health from environmental threats. This political initiative reflected an emerging consensus that living in a healthy, clean and safe environment was a basic human right, and that the disproportionate risk of toxic environments borne by poorer communities was an affront to social justice (Tamburlini *et al* 2002). That theme has been reflected in repeated international declarations, including the European Union's Environment and Health Strategy known as SCALE (Science, Children, Awareness, Legal instrument and Evaluation) and the Children's Environment and Health Action Plan for Europe. These statements widened the scope of environmental health beyond the traditional concerns of pollution and toxicity to include injuries, particularly to children and young people. This reflects an emerging view in some quarters that injuries – caused by the acute transfer of energy from the environment to human tissue – are an environmental health concern *par excellence* (Stone and Morris 2010).

Poorer countries stand to gain most from the implementation of more effective environmental health measures (Skolnik 2008). Among the highest priority actions that are necessary are:

➤ reducing outdoor air pollution through the introduction of unleaded fuel, tighter emission inspections of vehicles, and restrictions on the burning of refuse

➤ reducing indoor air pollution through the use of safer cooking devices and practices, improved ventilation, keeping children away from cooking areas, and restricting indoor tobacco smoking

➤ improving sanitation through the provision of more efficient latrines and sewer connections, and the enforcement of sanitary regulations

➤ providing clean domestic water through the more widespread use of house connection to the water supply, or well-maintained standpipes, combined with education about basic hygiene (mainly hand washing).

The growing green agenda

The environmentalist or 'green' agenda seeks to counter climate change, reduce dependence on motor vehicles, promote public transport, expand the consumption of healthy, locally produced food, and minimise social and health inequalities. It is another example of the interconnectedness of public health issues. Climate change is widely viewed by many commentators as the world's most serious and pressing public health priority. Advocates of immediate and drastic countermeasures are enthusiastic and vociferous, occasionally to the point of alarmism (Raziz 2010, Roberts 2011). A strident and quasi-religious zeal permeates many of their pronouncements (*see* Chapter 1) that could prove counterproductive.

Griffiths *et al* (2009) adopt a more sober attitude. They urge all healthcare practitioners to alert public and political opinion formers to the dangers of climate change, to seek to implement a global framework for reducing carbon emissions overall while permitting them to rise in poorer countries to assist their development, and to help develop a 'global social movement'. At the same time, they caution against adopting an excessively single-minded and obsessive focus on climate change, which is just one of many contemporary (though inter-related) global health challenges. Nevertheless, environmental interventions have the potential to achieve a wide range of beneficial outcomes, including the reduction or amelioration of poverty and social inequalities in health.

Priority 3: start early in the lifecourse to prevent disease and improve health

The argument that the various stages of the human life cycle are interconnected is so persuasive that it almost amounts to a truism. We have long known that growth and health throughout life are strongly influenced by genetics, maternal health, intrauterine development and the circumstances of birth, infancy and childhood. More recently, we have discovered that optimal brain development in early childhood is dependent on intellectual stimulation in the context of a warm, protective and nurturing emotional environment. Although all of these early exposures interact with later ones in complex and sometimes unpredictable ways, the major impact of early experience, positive and negative, from conception through to adolescence, is beyond question. Yet accepting the logic, based on decades of multidisciplinary research, of the desirability of intervening early in the lifecourse is one thing; producing convincing evidence of effective and significant long-term outcomes attributable to that intervention is quite another. Can we be confident that early intervention actually works? The answer has to be circumspect.

Early intervention to improve physical health

In terms of physical health, we have a formidable armamentarium of measures, based on reasonably solid research evidence, at our disposal. Primary prevention includes genetic counselling of families at risk of hereditary disease, fortification of flour with folate to prevent neural tube defects, reducing the exposure of the developing embryo and fetus to alcohol *in utero*, the promotion of exclusive breastfeeding of infants until the age of six months, fluoridation of drinking water to prevent dental caries, childhood immunisation programmes against common infections, anti-smoking policies and services to protect children from second-hand smoke, and the creation of safe environments to minimise the risk of injuries. Secondary prevention includes antenatal, neonatal and early childhood screening for the diagnosis of congenital anomalies (such as hypothyroidism and phenylketonuria) or remediable sensory deficits, the use of safety equipment (such as car seat restraints or bicycle helmets) to reduce the severity of injuries, and the implementation of child protection measures where abuse or neglect is suspected. Tertiary prevention includes the provision of aids (such as wheelchairs to enhance the mobility of disabled children), and the prescription of long-term prophylactic medication (such as inhalers to reduce the frequency and severity of asthma attacks). Note that these measures are frequently 'individualistic' – that is, neither purely population based nor environmental in nature – and involve what some public health practitioners might regard, with a degree of unease, as routine clinical care. But access to basic medical care for parents (especially mothers) and children can prevent or ameliorate threats to health and development and ensure early diagnosis and treatment when necessary.

Early intervention to improve mental health and social outcomes
Interventions to promote mental health, cognitive development and positive long-term health, educational and social outcomes are far from straightforward and are currently being intensively researched. Early, intensive support for parents, provided through skilled home visiting, appears to be effective in improving several health and social outcomes, as do high-quality early education programmes. Geddes *et al* (2010), in reviewing the world literature on interventions designed to promote child development and health, concluded that early intervention programmes can help reduce the impact of social disadvantage, and that significant improvements in all domains of child development, school achievement, delinquency and crime prevention, and life success have been demonstrated. They found that successful interventions often adopted a mixed, two-generation approach – that is, a combination of centre- and home-based programmes with both child and parent components. No single approach has, as yet, been shown to offer a 'magic bullet'.

The research evidence is unclear on whether universal or targeted approaches work best. The greatest effects are certainly found in programmes that target those at highest social risk but that could simply reflect the nature of the populations selected for study – universal interventions are harder and more expensive to evaluate than targeted ones. Most experts favour a combined approach whereby universal services are supplemented by intensive interventions for those thought to have greatest need, however defined. Although developmental (including IQ) gains seem greatest in early childhood, improved academic achievement persists over longer periods and leads to better outcomes in adult life. Well-evaluated generic or 'horizontal' programmes are rare. Exceptions include the Nurse Family Partnership (Olds *et al* 2007), the Chicago Parent-Child Centers (Karoly *et al* 2005), the Positive Parenting Programme or Triple P (Sanders *et al* 2003),

Incredible Years (Webster-Stratton 1998) and Sure Start (Melhuish *et al* 2008), all of which have reported positive outcomes from various locations.

Politics of early intervention

Early intervention as a public health strategy is beginning to win strong political support around the world. In the UK, for example, Allen and Smith (2008), two members of Parliament from opposing parties, secured non-partisan endorsement from their party leaders for the principle of an early years strategy (though there may have a partial retreat in the wake of the budgetary cuts to local authorities in 2011–12). Advocates of early intervention emphasise that reducing expenditure on children is a false economy. Although the initial financial investments are substantial, the economic returns appear to be many times greater with benefit to cost ratios ranging from 2:1 to 17:1 depending on the programme (Karoly *et al* 2005). Among the various measures Allen and Smith proposed was the release of public funds for early intervention from some of the 'massive future savings' from improved outcomes, particularly in disadvantaged groups, likely to accrue through such investment (see Chapter 3). The alternative, they argued, is to take ever-increasing amounts of taxation from the public to deal with the impact of failing to intervene early.

All of these measures must be calibrated to meet epidemiologically assessed local and national needs and to take account of the broader geographical, political, economic and cultural context. Affluent countries may be in a better position to focus on childhood screening and the promotion of neuropsychological development than poorer ones as the latter are still grappling with a large burden of malnutrition, diarrhoea and infections. Ultimately, however, all children have the same basic needs, albeit to a varying degree. The principle of equity requires that we recognise that all human beings have an equal right to fulfil their potential for health and wellbeing. Where there is need, and an available evidence-based response, there is an obligation on public health services to meet it regardless of the place or setting in which it happens to be located.

Priority 4: adopt a horizontal strategic framework for global public health

Need for better collaboration

Collaboration and co-operation are essential to strategic development in global public health. Among the many reasons for this are:

➤ increasing globalisation, with all the risks and opportunities associated with international travel, migration, trade and information exchange

➤ the value of sharing knowledge about efficacious approaches to health improvement, disease prevention and treatment

➤ the need to set technical standards for interventions such as vaccines

➤ a recognition that some health threats, such as pollution and infection, are no respecters of national boundaries

➤ the practical and ethical imperatives of confronting inequality whereby stronger, richer countries can assist weaker, poorer ones.

There are many outstanding examples of collaboration that have yielded real and lasting benefits. The most spectacular case in recent times was the eradication of smallpox by 1980, perhaps the WHO's finest hour. All three elements of public health – diagnosis, treatment and follow-up – worked synergistically and effectively. The inspirational value of this success should not be underestimated; if smallpox can be defeated, other diseases and problems can too.

Yet simple exhortation to collaborate is never sufficient. People need tangible incentives, whether these appear as duties in their job descriptions or as working targets that will virtually ensure collaboration with other sectors and colleagues. The most effective way of guaranteeing collaboration is to hardwire it into the way organisations are created. Function flows from structure. When an organisation is structured to reflect its collaborative functions, a co-operative mode of working will inevitably emerge. This seems to hold true whatever the size of the organisation or whether its remit is local or national. Equally, international co-operation is bound to flow more freely from a global infrastructure that is specifically designed to facilitate it.

Need for global infrastructure

Infrastructures may be intellectual or organisational. International agencies such as the WHO have tried hard to develop both in the public health field. Greater progress has been made in creating intellectual (or philosophical) infrastructures though much remains to be done in both areas. The Ottawa Charter and similar declarations have been instrumental in offering an inspirational vision but are insufficient in the absence of a comprehensive and detailed strategic plan – an explicit set of goals, objectives and actions to enable the vision to be realised. The WHO should strive to develop and obtain a consensus around a comprehensive, horizontal plan; the proposed global public health strategy in the Appendix is one possible model. Once created, that intellectual infrastructure (the strategic plan along with the available knowledge, skills and personnel) can then be deployed for implementation, evaluation and future planning. All of that is possible with minimal resources allied to clear-sighted and determined senior management teams working within and across international agencies. But the agencies themselves are not always fit for purpose and may be in need of major reform.

Role of international agencies

A plethora of actors currently occupy the global public health stage (Box 10.4). On paper, the UN, World Bank, International Monetary Fund (IMF) and WHO – the global civil service – are well placed to promote international collabo-

---

BOX 10.4 *Some key global health agencies*

United Nations
➤ World Health Organization
➤ UN Development Program
➤ UN Fund for Population Activities
➤ UN Children's Fund (UNICEF)
➤ International Monetary Fund

Development banks and agencies
➤ World Bank
➤ African, Asian and Inter-American development banks
➤ National aid agencies (e.g. United States Agency for International Development)

Other agencies
➤ Foundations (e.g. Bill and Melinda Gates Foundation)
➤ NGOs (e.g. Medecins Sans Frontières, OXFAM)
➤ Special programmes and partnerships (e.g. Global Alliance for Vaccines and Immunisation, Malaria Vaccine Initiative)

---

ration in public health, to undertake strategic planning and to forge strong links between centres of excellence and underserved countries. In practice, their performance falls short of their ambition. Arguably the most successful (and respected) of these is the WHO.

The WHO was established in 1948 by the United Nations. Its declared objective was (and is) to promote 'the attainment by all peoples of the highest possible level of health', health being defined holistically (*see* Introduction). According to its website (www.who.int/en/index.html):

> WHO is the directing and coordinating authority for health within the United Nations system. It is responsible for providing leadership on global health matters, shaping the health research agenda, setting norms and standards, articulating evidence-based policy options, providing technical support to countries and monitoring and assessing health trends.

The WHO's key roles are advocacy, consensus building, knowledge sharing, disease surveillance, setting global technical standards, and leading or supporting international agreements and initiatives. It has limited financial resources and is governed through the annual World Health Assembly (WHA) that determines WHO policy, approves the budget and appoints the Director General.

The WHO is thus essentially at the mercy of the WHA and its sometimes dysfunctional political processes.

Some of the WHO's most notable successes have been in the field of infectious disease surveillance and control, especially the eradication of smallpox and its near-eradication of polio. Others include its encouragement of breastfeeding, its campaigns on childhood immunisations, and its efforts to control tobacco consumption. It was instrumental in launching the Health for All initiative and the Ottawa Charter, and in supporting the creation of international partnerships such as the Global Fund to Fight against AIDS, TB and Malaria. In recent times, the WHO has faced many serious challenges to its authority and integrity. Among its failings may be counted excessive bureaucracy, lack of accountability, and distortion of policies through politicisation, uncertain leadership, internal feuding and a perceived decline in effectiveness. The disappointing results of international efforts to reduce the incidence and prevalence of TB and malaria have been especially damaging to the WHO's reputation.

At times, the WHO seems besieged by criticism from all sides. In some instances, such as the HIV/AIDS pandemic, it has been accused of complacency; in others, such as the H1N1 (swine flu) scare, it has allegedly over-reacted. Some of its more strident critics have accused the agency of weak governance, secrecy and undeclared conflicts of interest; others have invoked the spectre of conspiracies (Cohen and Carter 2010). For the WHO, operating in the full glare of international publicity and subjected to conflicting political pressures, this is arguably a no-win situation. By its nature, the work the WHO performs is often controversial and liable to be judged excessively harshly.

To sum up: for all their shortcomings, the United Nations and related agencies have generally been a force for good in seeking to promote strategic thinking in global health and, in particular, to address the plight of mothers and children. Since the Second World War, several UN agencies have played a leading role in collaborative international activities aimed at improving population health in general and maternal and child health in particular. Their considerable achievements, when set against their failings, should be acknowledged.

Priority 5: improve global health data

Better quality data are urgently needed

Making an accurate diagnosis depends on having access to all the relevant information. Epidemiologists struggle with inadequate data wherever they work. The ongoing Global Burden of Disease study is severely hamstrung by these constraints. The scale of the problem is staggering: Setel *et al* (2007) estimate that only one-third of the 57 million annual deaths and two-thirds of the 128 million annual births in the world are registered. That means that many millions of people, especially those (around half of the total) who live in rural areas, may be born, live out their lives and die without leaving behind any official record that they ever existed. That amounts to a barely recognised international scandal that requires urgent remedy. In the circumstances, it is remarkable that the GBD study has been able to generate as much information as it has.

Even where deaths and their causes are recorded, whether in affluent or poor countries, the validity of this information is largely unknown. Some countries (including large ones such as China and India) employ sample registration systems to generate vital statistics of questionable validity. And other key dimensions of the disease burden, such as incidence, prevalence, morbidity and disability, are equally unsatisfactory. There are exceptions. Where national or local statistical agencies, disease registries, laboratory surveillance systems and periodic population surveys are well run and adequately funded, better quality data are available. Generally speaking, though, the global information landscape can only be described as bleak.

Countries that fail to maintain adequate civil registration systems are actually in breach of their commitments to legal instruments including the Convention on the Rights of the Child, the International Covenant on Civil and Political Rights, and the Convention Relating to the Rights of Stateless Persons (AbouZahr et al 2010). This obligation is neither supported nor enforced by international agencies. The support required is twofold – technical and financial. A combination of longitudinal population surveillance supplemented by verbal autopsy is one technical solution, albeit an interim one until sufficient investment is forthcoming. The scale of financing that would be required to pursue this course is relatively trivial – around 10 cents per person annually in Africa, according to the MDG Africa Steering Group. The investment would reap rich dividends, not only for epidemiologists but for the countries themselves given that data-driven public health is so important for economic development. On a more positive note, the MDGs have at least exposed the huge gaps in health statistics in poorer countries. That has prompted at least one encouraging new initiative – the creation of the Institute for Health Metrics and Evaluation at the University of Washington, Seattle, funded by the Bill and Melinda Gates Foundation.

Using available data more effectively

Calling for better data on global health is sometimes used as a delaying tactic, a figleaf for lack of action. In fact, a vast quantity of data (admittedly of variable quality) already exists and could be used more effectively for research, advocacy and monitoring. That in itself poses a challenge – how to analyse and present the available data in a manner that is comprehensible to policy makers, practitioners and the public. Ideally, the data should be presented in a form that describes both the epidemiological profile of a country and the policy response to it. Beaglehole and Bonita (2009) propose an elegant solution: a 'public health scorecard' as a means of benchmarking national responses to five groups of population health problems (maternal, neonatal and child health, infectious diseases, chronic diseases, environmental changes and social determinants). The responses would be documented across four dimensions (leadership, infrastructure, evidence for action and health systems). The scorecard would identify areas in which the performance of global public health needs strengthening. Further development of this idea would presumably require the support of the WHO and other organisations, notably the Institute of Health Metrics and Evaluation.

Health data are often presented in a format that non-health professionals and policy makers find unhelpful. Because 'healthy public policies', as called for by the Ottawa Charter, require non-health sectors to take a degree of responsibility for public health, health information must convey clearer messages to those sectors to enable them to respond appropriately. Parker *et al* (2010) assert that a gap exists between available information and the way data are framed for non-health policy makers. They propose an agenda for research into the exploitation of epidemiological data for the advocacy of health-promoting policies. More sophisticated analyses are required to present and disseminate data for this purpose, and these should highlight the social and environmental determinants of health, and quantify the burden of disease that is avoidable by policy.

Priority 6: boost public health capacity

Throughout history, the world has suffered from a deficiency of personnel, skills, education and training in public health. Resources for public health training, especially in poor countries, are always overstretched. Today, the position is too serious to ignore. Any future investment in public health capacity building will have to come predominantly from wealthy countries where public health education is well established. Schools of public health have proliferated across Europe and North America in recent years though many of these are committed primarily to research rather than teaching.

In the past, too many doctors regarded public health as a low-status, financially unrewarding and intellectually undemanding specialty. That perception is rapidly changing. Medical schools are becoming more receptive to the teaching of public health to future doctors though in many places traditionalists continue to hold senior academic positions and remain stubbornly resistant to change. The old rigid division between clinical and public health education is slowly being dismantled. Pioneering 'community-oriented' medical schools, such as McMaster in Canada, Maastricht in The Netherlands and Beer Sheva in Israel, have demonstrated that it is possible to integrate clinical and public health education given sufficient motivation and enthusiasm (Stone 2000).

At postgraduate level, the development of accreditation systems, based on assessments conducted either by examination or peer review, is essential for the setting and maintenance of competence in public health wherever it is provided and by whomever it is practised. In resource-poor countries, where Masters of Public Health courses are especially thin on the ground, one solution might be to exploit new educational technologies such as open-access online resources (Heller *et al* 2007). Several websites are leading the way in providing free postgraduate lectures and other educational materials for public health students worldwide. These include the Epidemiology Supercourse (www.pitt.edu/~super1), MERLOT (www.merlot.org), the People's Open Access Educational Initiative (http://peoples-uni.org/) and the Development Gateway (http://topics.developmentgateway.org/openeducation).

FROM STRATEGIC PLANNING TO IMPLEMENTATION

Good strategic planning is something of a paradox. Although its content appears to be the product of an intellectual exercise, the process of generating that content is a pragmatic one that has to be rooted in reality. A strategy is judged by its practicality rather than by its creativity. If the strategy appears irrelevant to stakeholders, it will fail. Yet even if the strategy secures widespread support, success is far from guaranteed. Once a strategy has been developed and endorsed, and its implications agreed – whether in terms of the 60 action points or six priorities shown in the Appendix or some other formulation – the really hard work of implementation begins. That in turn throws up a new set of challenges, none of which is entirely inseparable from the strategy itself. Meeting those challenges is the topic of the next chapter.

REFERENCES

AbouZahr C, Gooogly L, Stevens G. Better data needed: everyone agrees, but no one wants to pay. *Lancet.* 2010; **375**: 619–21.

Allen G, Smith ID. *Good Parents, Great Kids, Better Citizens.* London: Centre for Social Justice and Smith Institute; 2008.

Beaglehole T, Bonita R. A scorecard for assessing progress in global public health. *J Epidemiol Commun Health.* 2009; **63**: 507–8.

Bellagio Study Group on Child Survival. How many child deaths can we prevent this year? *Lancet.* 2003; **362**: 65–71.

Cohen D, Carter P. WHO and the pandemic flu 'conspiracies.' *BMJ.* 2010; **340**: c2912.

Collier P. *The Bottom Billion. Why the poorest countries are failing and what can be done about it.* New York: Oxford University Press; 2008.

Geddes R, Haw S, Frank J. *Interventions for Promoting Early Child Development for Health: an environmental scan with special reference to Scotland.* Edinburgh: Scottish Collaboration for Public Health Research and Policy; 2010.

Griffiths J, Rao M, Adshead F, *et al. The Health Practitioner's Guide to Climate Change: diagnosis and cure.* London: Earthscan; 2009.

Guo B, Harstall C. *For Which Strategies of Suicide Prevention is There Evidence of Effectiveness?* Copenhagen: WHO Regional Office for Europe; 2004.

Heller RF, Chongsuvivatwong V, Hailegeogios S, *et al.* Capacity-building for public health: http://peoples-uni.org. *Bull World Health Organ.* 2007; **85**: 930–4.

Karoly LA, Kilburn MR, Cannon JS. *Early Childhood Interventions: proven results, future promise.* Santa Monica, CA: RAND Corporation; 2005.

Mann JJ, Apter A, Bertolote J, *et al.* Suicide prevention strategies: a systematic review. *JAMA.* 2005; **294**: 2064–74.

McVeigh C, Hughes K, Bellis MA, Reed E, Ashton JR, Syed Q. *Violent Britain: people, prevention and public health.* Liverpool: John Moores University; 2005.

Melhuish EC, Belsky J, Leyland AH, *et al.* Effects of fully-established Sure Start local programmes on 3-year-old children and their families living in England: a quasi-experimental observational study. *Lancet.* 2008; **372**: 1641–7.

Olds DL, Sadler L, Kitzman H. Programs for parents of infants and toddlers: recent evidence from randomised trials. *Child Psychol Psychiatry.* 2007; **48**: 355–91.

Parker LA, Lumbreras B, Hernandez-Aguado I. Health information and advocacy for 'Health in All Policies': a research agenda. *J Epidemiol Commun Health.* 2010; **64**: 114–16.

Peden M, Scurfield R, Sleet D, *et al. World Report on Road Traffic Injury Prevention.* Geneva: World Health Organization; 2004.

Raziz DV. The risk of a sixth mass extinction of life and the role of medicine. *J R Soc Med.* 2010; **103**: 473–4.

Roberts I. Fat chance for Cancun. *J R Soc Med.* 2011; **104**: 43–4.

Sachs J. *The End of Poverty.* London: Penguin Books; 2005.

Sanders MR, Markie-Dadds C, Turner KMT. Theoretical, scientific and clinical foundations of the Triple P Positive Parenting Programme: a population approach to the promotion of parenting competence. *Parenting Res Pract Monograph.* 2003; **1**: 1–21.

Setel PW, Macfarlane SB, Szreter S, *et al.* A scandal of invisibility: making everyone count by counting everyone. *Lancet.* 2007; **370**: 1726–35.

Skolnik R. *Essentials of Global Health.* Sudbury, MA: Jones and Bartlett Learning; 2008.

Smith KR, Corvalan CF, Kjellstrom T. How much global ill health is attributable to environmental factors? *Epidemiology.* 1999; **10**: 573.

Stone DH. Public health in the undergraduate medical curriculum – can we achieve integration? *J Eval Clin Pract.* 2000; **6**: 9–14.

Stone DH, Morris GP. Injury prevention: a strategic priority for environmental health? *Public Health.* 2010; **124**: 559–64.

Sustainable Development Commission. *Sustainable Development: the key to tackling health inequalities.* London: Sustainable Development Commission; 2010.

Tamburlini G, von Ehrenstein OS, Bertollini R, editors. *Children's Health and Environment: a review of evidence.* Copenhagen: World Health Organization Regional Office for Europe; 2002.

United Nations. *Every Woman, Every Child: global strategy for women's and children's health.* 2010. www.un.org/sg/hf/global strategy commitments.pdf

Webster-Stratton C. Preventing conduct problems in Head Start children: strengthening parent competencies. *J Consult Clin Psychol.* 1998; **66**: 715–30.

World Health Organization. *Global Status Report on Non-Communicable Diseases 2010.* Geneva: World Health Organization; 2011.

World Health Organization Framework Convention on Tobacco Control. 2003. www.who.int/fctc/text_download/en/index.html

World Health Organization/John Moores University. *Violence Prevention – the evidence.* Geneva: World Health Organization; 2009.

Section 2 summary

Because we are confronting a global challenge, we need to mount a global response. The response should comprise measures that include the development of a global public health action plan or strategy.

Some strategic elements already exist in the texts of international agreements such as the Ottawa Charter (1986) and the Millennium Declaration (2000). Both of those initiatives have been extremely influential in setting the agenda for global public health. While these and other international endeavours are all important in their own right, they need to be integrated into a single, horizontal strategic framework of a kind that currently does not exist.

There are two distinct, if connected, aspects of strategy development. The first is the final statement that sets out the roadmap for producing change. The second is the process itself. Rather than being merely a means to an end, the process of strategy development contains within it the seeds of the strategy's success or failure.

Here is one of many possible versions of a public health mission statement for our time.

> To embrace, at a global level, a model of public health that is holistic in scope and aspires to influence the health of populations with a view to:
> - improving and protecting health and wellbeing (physical, mental and social)
> - preventing ill health (and the risk of ill health), disability and suffering
> - reducing health inequalities between genders, races, social groups, communities and countries
> - nurturing an ecologically sustainable environment for future generations.

I have attempted to articulate five *key principles* that should inform a horizontal global public health strategy (*see* the Appendix).
1 Embrace a holistic view of health and disease on which to base public health responses.
2 Apply a pragmatic evidence-based approach to public health policy making and practice.
3 Adopt a lifecourse perspective on public health analysis and intervention.

4 Create efficient and transparent governance processes for public health action.

5 Strive for a strategic overview of public health policy making and practice.

The three top priorities that I have selected for immediate horizontal strategic action are:

➤ work with others to eliminate absolute poverty and ameliorate relative poverty

➤ start early in the lifecourse to prevent disease and improve health

➤ focus on creating a healthy, safe and sustainable environment.

The three top priorities that I have selected for improving the infrastructure are:

➤ adopt a horizontal strategic framework for global public health while continuing to deliver vertical interventions

➤ improve routine health data completeness and quality

➤ boost public health capacity in the form of personnel, skills and resources.

SECTION 3
Follow-up

CHAPTER 11

Ensuring implementation

When a doctor prescribes a treatment for a patient, there is no guarantee that the patient will comply. There are numerous possible reasons for this. The patient may not understand the nature of the treatment or have anxieties about side-effects. Or access to a pharmacist may be obstructed by cost or distance. Or the patient may simply mistrust doctors or suspect their motives. Most of these difficulties may be overcome by the application of skilled clinical advice, careful and detailed explanation, the investment of staff time in allaying the patient's fears, in responding to questions, and by creating mechanisms for doctor–patient liaison and follow-up.

Without stretching the clinical analogy too far, it is possible to view 'public health prescribing' in a similar light. Compliance with international, national or local public health strategies cannot be taken for granted but can be facilitated in various ways: capacity building, promoting better communication, networking and collaboration, allocating sufficient resources in the form of personnel and finance, incorporating robust performance management systems, and creating an effective administrative infrastructure for the smooth running of the various components of the public health system. Giving careful thought, at an early stage, to the processes that are involved in implementation and monitoring will reap dividends.

GOOD INTENTIONS ARE NOT ENOUGH

A strategic policy statement or plan amounts to little more than an assertion of good intentions, however carefully crafted. Merely stating what you want to achieve and how you are going to go about it is no guarantee of success. Articulating principles, setting goals, developing a plan – these are all necessary but insufficient steps towards achieving the vision of better population health. In itself, strategic planning – however comprehensive and thoughtful – changes nothing. Without ensuring that the plans are actually implemented in the manner intended, the entire process risks becoming a sterile academic exercise. Worse, it may undermine public and professional confidence in the strategy and may discredit the agency or individuals attempting to promote it. Paradoxically, the planning process, by raising expectations that are then dashed, may thereby become part of the problem rather than part of the solution.

How can the implementation of a public health strategy be guaranteed? The short answer is that it can't, at least not within a democratic setting. We can, however, optimise the likelihood of implementation if we create appropriate and properly resourced delivery vehicles. In global public health terms, that means we need to develop and refine a global public health infrastructure (*see* Chapter 10) that works in tandem with other international agencies (including non-governmental organisations (NGOs)), national and local governments.

While considering how to create the most effective delivery vehicles, it is worth taking several preliminary steps to oil the wheels of implementation. These include setting priorities (which diseases or actions will be addressed first), defining specific responsibilities (designating leadership and operational roles), describing the resources and skills needed (finance and personnel), and creating mechanisms for monitoring and evaluation (of the process of policy development and its implementation).

CONTEXT OF PUBLIC HEALTH PRACTICE

For a strategy to succeed, it has to be driven to the point of implementation by a committed individual, team or agency. Allocating sufficient resources to the task will be a crucial determinant of success, as will the ability to work with a range of colleagues outside the formal public health sphere. The organisational context of public health practice may either facilitate or obstruct such a mode of working. Holland and Stewart (1998) suggested that public health practitioners have to be able to do three things to fulfil their role effectively:
➤ to be forthright in their advocacy of health improvement programmes and strategies
➤ to control the budget for public health activities, both in the short and long term
➤ to assume a clearly identifiable role in helping to influence both the health sector and other relevant agencies.

Those three requirements – advocacy, resources and leadership – are most likely to be fulfilled within an 'arm's length' organisation rather than one that is embedded within the bureaucratic setting of government or the healthcare system. Unfortunately, that degree of independence and autonomy is simply a chimera for most public health staff.

ORGANISING TO DELIVER

Developing appropriate organisational structures to facilitate implementation is crucial. As mentioned in previous chapters, merely exhorting organisations, departments, groups or individuals to work together is usually doomed to failure. Internal rather than external agendas will always take priority. Unless interagency working is written into job plans, with unambiguous lines of managerial responsibility and accountability, it is unlikely to happen. Collaborative, intersectoral working rarely occurs spontaneously. A more effective approach is to recognise that function flows from structure and to establish organisational entities to promote joint working. Such structures need not be rigid and permanent – short-life task forces can prove highly effective – but they should exist. In parallel with an effort to develop fresh strategic thinking, governments and international agencies must work to secure sustained policy commitment to multisectoral health improvement led at the highest level by senior political leaders and officials. They will be better placed to rise to the challenge if adequate administrative structures and resources are made available to support them.

In the past, many public health commentators were somewhat dismissive of the role of healthcare systems in health improvement efforts. They pointed to the strong epidemiological evidence that increasing life expectancy in the 19th century in the industrialised world was attributable to better housing, nutrition, water supplies and sewage disposal. That view has begun to change. Modern healthcare systems almost invariably define their primary aim as health improvement. Working in tandem with other sectors, healthcare systems are increasingly recognised as a key element in national and global public health initiatives. Sharma and Atri (2010) go further:

> Most of the recent global reduction in mortality and morbidity secondary to infectious diseases has been attributed to the fact that countries around the globe have built effective health systems that streamline the care delivery process.

Immunisation illustrates this point. It is one of the few medical interventions, largely organised and delivered by healthcare systems, whose benefits unequivocally outweigh its costs (Logan and Bedford 1995). Ensuring the highest possible level of coverage is essential to the effectiveness of an immunisation programme and this is best achieved by exploiting the routine contacts that people have with primary care services. Staff training, to increase awareness of guidelines and to nurture enthusiasm and skills, is the responsibility of the healthcare system. Accurate record keeping designed to check and respond to the immunisation status of patients is another important element that lies within the orbit of healthcare system management, as do the related activities of performance audit and programme monitoring.

Probably the greatest challenges facing healthcare systems derive from their need to secure adequate funding, and to invest available resources in the most effective and efficient manner. Various models of healthcare have been tried, ranging from wholly government-funded systems to wholly private ones and all varieties in between. The most popular approach seems to be the 'mixed economy' in which public and private agencies work in partnership. For the poorest countries of the world, resources are so scarce that no form of mass healthcare provision of any kind is feasible.

POLITICS AND PUBLIC HEALTH

There is no escaping the fact that all public health has a political component. That is inevitable and even desirable. Only political action can achieve the large-scale shift in resources or legislation that many public health problems require. If public health practitioners adopt a posture of lofty detachment from politics, they will risk accusations of naivety at best and hypocrisy at worst.

Political awareness of public health issues has many dimensions. It includes an understanding of how the public perceives particular diseases or counter-measures through the lens of media reporting. It also involves an appreciation of the most effective way to ensure that public health measures are integrated into political programmes that have to take account of competing priorities. When they grasp the nuances of the political context, public health professionals are in a far better position to exploit opportunities for intervention and overcome obstacles. Politicians are highly sensitive to public expectations relating to a specific problem or cluster of concerns, particularly when these are translated into media campaigns, social movements, lobby groups or voting behaviour (Oliver 2006).

But there are inherent risks associated with the politics of public health. One policy or strategy may overlap with or even contradict another, leading to duplication, misunderstanding, tension or conflict between departments or individuals. A major problem arises when politicisation – the manipulation of non-political activities for political purposes – intrudes. Global efforts to implement public health policies depend on the integration of the supranational infrastructure with non-partisan political forces in a way that achieves global public health objectives. The UN experience is not an altogether happy one in this regard. The 'one country, one vote' system of UN and World Health Association governance is immaculately democratic in theory but in practice reduces consensus making to the lowest common denominator. At the same time, it exposes these institutions to the vagaries of block voting by groups of countries who, for whatever reason, wish to obstruct discussion on particular issues, such as women's rights, climate change or conflict resolution, or to divert attention away from sensitive issues towards (often spurious) 'root causes' of health, poverty and related problems.

Even when international consensus is secured, the implementation of strategic plans is dependent on mutual trust and co-operation between supranational agencies and national, or even local, authorities. National governments are ultimately responsible for policy and practice in their own countries, albeit with the encouragement of international agencies. All are beset by their own internal rivalries and conflicts, and all struggle with implementation. Because every set of circumstances is unique, teasing out generalisable lessons from the national experience of particular countries is difficult.

FIVE NATIONAL CASE STUDIES

There is great heterogeneity across national governments in the way they have attempted to deliver public health interventions to their residents. Yet despite their differences, they all share the same over-riding goal – to improve population health. We should be able to learn a great deal, including identifying some general features of effective implementation, from both their successes and failures.

Below are five thumbnail sketches of the way in which five contrasting countries have addressed the task of improving the health status of their populations. The selection has not been based on their representativeness but because they illustrate some valuable principles. Two of the countries are affluent western European ones, one is an emerging east European economic power, and two are very large developing countries.

The United Kingdom

The National Health Service, created in 1948 and free at the point of use to all UK citizens, has explicitly articulated health improvement as well as healthcare objectives. Better population health has been a policy objective of every government regardless of its political hue. Health authorities, along with some specialised nationwide agencies, employ multidisciplinary public health consultants and health promotion officers. Prior to 1972, the public health workforce was mainly located within local authorities, to which they seem likely to revert (at least in England) in the future. Despite periodic attempts to develop both comprehensive and disorder-specific national public health strategies, successive British governments have struggled to prioritise prevention in the face of ever-increasing demands for expensive therapies and services (Lock and Sim 2009).

Despite these obstacles, UK public health has achieved some outstanding successes, such as the high coverage of child immunisation and screening programmes, the legal requirement to wear seatbelts in cars, and the introduction of legislation to outlaw smoking in enclosed public spaces. There have also been serious disappointments, perhaps the most notable being the low level of wellbeing of UK children compared to other affluent countries, and the long-standing failure to reduce social inequalities in health. Some of this may be attributed to two specific failings – the absence of a coherent population health strategy, and an obsession with individual lifestyle factors to the near-exclusion of environmental and other important determinants of health.

Sweden

Sweden has long been envied in public health circles for its remarkable record of health improvement, lengthening life expectancy and progress towards social equity. The country is often placed at or near the top of international league tables of good health and wellbeing, even within the small group of high-achieving elite nations that comprise Scandinavia. These achievements reflect several interacting factors: sustained economic prosperity, a culture of collectivism and a sophisticated public health infrastructure. Other key advantages are the country's investment in high-quality routine health information and epidemiological research, and a strong commitment by successive governments to properly funded, well-co-ordinated public health policies and programmes. Intervention measures frequently straddle individual and population-based approaches, take account of familial, community and environmental factors, and are often specifically targeted at parents, children and young people. Both the public health community and the main political parties appear to recognise the need to address 'upstream' health determinants, such as emotional health, social capital and community resilience, as well as more 'downstream' disease and social outcomes.

While this scenario may seem to outside observers an idyllic one, Sweden nevertheless grapples with many of the same public health problems as those afflicting other affluent countries: rising rates of chronic disease and disability due to an ageing population, the growing impact of the obesity pandemic, and persistent or even widening health inequalities between social and ethnic groups (Wall *et al* 2009).

Russia

The transition from communism to democracy in Russia and the Soviet bloc countries has been a mixed blessing. While liberating for individuals and harbouring the promise of a better quality of life for many of its citizens in the future, its impact seems to have been largely negative from a public health perspective, at least in the short term. The political and social upheavals of the 1990s, combined with a historical legacy of outmoded, inefficient and sometimes corrupt public health practices, led to a sharp deterioration in population health, including a drop in life expectancy. This occurred at a time when western European residents were enjoying substantial improvements in health.

McKee (2009) attributed the rise in deaths in early middle age, particularly in men, to the destructive role of alcohol, especially when it is so easily accessible as cheap non-beverage liquids. Alcohol, when consumed excessively, can damage fetal development and is causally associated with numerous diseases (including cirrhosis of the liver and mental illness) and injuries (including road casualties, suicides and homicides). The high prevalence of smoking and a diet rich in saturated fats are responsible for the unfavourable Russian death rates from cardiovascular disease and cancer.

Both the healthcare and public health systems were (and remain) ill equipped to respond to these challenges. Despite a reasonably high-quality system of vital statistics, epidemiological data are seldom analysed and presented in a manner that highlights trends or problems. Practitioners lack the skills or organisational support to implement effective countermeasures. Public health capacity, in general, is insufficient to address the needs of the population though a few newly established schools of public health are making inroads into the skills gap.

China

China epitomises the plight of countries undergoing the demographic and epidemiological transitions (Lee and Lv 2009). Life expectancy doubled from 35 years before 1949 to 71 years for men and 75 years for women in 2005. Despite the one-child policy introduced in the 1970s, the population also doubled in size in that period. The older infectious diseases are giving way to newer ones, including HIV/AIDS and tuberculosis (TB). The rapidly ageing population has propelled chronic diseases, injuries and mental health problems much higher up the national agenda. As in western countries, the main causes of death are cardiovascular diseases, cancer and chronic respiratory diseases. The pattern of smoking prevalence diverges markedly from western countries in that it is over 50% in men while very low (3%) in women. Other chronic disease risk factors causing concern include physical inactivity, obesity and high blood pressure. Social and urban-rural inequalities in health are increasing.

Although prevention has a hallowed place in Chinese culture and traditional medical practice, many commentators view the public health system as currently unfit for purpose. The national and regional infrastructure has received considerable investment in recent years but remains fragile and beset by enormous problems: information systems are fragmented and unco-ordinated; the workforce is inadequately trained and disproportionately concentrated in urban areas; public health education is neglected; interventions are excessively dependent on laws, ordinances and codes; and management practices are outdated and inefficient. Having said that, the future may be much brighter. China is still undergoing rapid change in all spheres of life and the public health system will be no exception.

India

In common with other developing countries, India is undergoing the epidemiological transition from a disease pattern dominated by infectious and nutritional diseases to one in which chronic (especially cardiovascular) diseases, injuries and mental illness are becoming increasingly prominent (Thakker and Reddy 2009). Life expectancy has increased over the past half-century and fertility has declined. Regional variations in health indicators, such as infant mortality rates, are striking, with Kerala and Tamil Nadu comparing favourably with many middle-income countries. The unfinished agenda of communicable diseases includes malaria (which resurfaced in the 1970s after a prolonged period of decline), TB and HIV/AIDS. Maternal mortality remains relatively high and child immunisation rates are extremely variable. Chronic disorders, such as cardiovascular diseases, cancer and diabetes, are on the rise as are mental disorders and injuries. Spending on healthcare and public health is one of the lowest in the world and there is a chronic shortage of skilled personnel, many of whom emigrate to pursue careers abroad.

Nevertheless, there have been major public health successes including the eradication of smallpox, a steep decline in polio incidence and the positive impact of family planning services. The Integrated Child Development Service (launched in 1974) and the National Rural Health Mission (launched in 2005) appear to have improved nutritional status, immunisation uptake and perhaps primary school performance. The main barriers to further progress include inadequate financial and human resource allocation, inequitable access to healthcare and preventive services (partly due to growing privatisation), and a disjointed public health infrastructure. Like China, India's rapid economic growth should ensure that more resources are channelled into the public health infrastructure in the future.

COMMON THEMES?

Can we draw any general lessons about the implementation of public health strategies and measures from these five examples? From the above accounts, it is clear that every country is unique yet some common themes are discernible. All face the consequences of changing demography and, in the case of the poorer countries, the epidemiological transition. All are committed to improving population health and the reduction in inequalities in health through the launching of well-co-ordinated horizontal and vertical strategies. All recognise the importance of generating and allocating sufficient resources to support the development of a range of systems and activities. Among the most crucial of these are good-quality health information systems, centrally led but locally delivered strategic planning, the creation of a robust public health infrastructure staffed by a skilled and well-motivated workforce, the implementation of evidence-based interventions and the systematic monitoring of outcomes.

A shortlist of the key attributes of a successful public health delivery system might therefore include:

➤ availability of reliable and relevant data on population health
➤ professional and political leadership in public health
➤ coherent planning linked to well-managed, evidence-based frontline programmes
➤ allocation of adequate financial and human resources
➤ deployment of practitioners with appropriate skills
➤ development of capacity through education and training
➤ co-ordination of healthcare and preventive services
➤ careful monitoring of performance and outcomes.

The last bullet point emphasises the need to incorporate evaluation into every strategy and implementation plan. The topic is of such over-riding importance that it deserves a chapter of its own.

REFERENCES

Holland WW, Stewart S. *Public Health: the vision and the challenge*. London: Nuffield Trust; 1998.

Lee L, Lv J. Public health in China: history and contemporary challenges. In: Beaglehole R, Bonita R, editors. *Global Public Health: a new era*. Oxford: Oxford University Press; 2009. pp.185–207.

Lock K, Sim F. Public health in the United Kingdom. In: Beaglehole R, Bonita R, editors. *Global Public Health: a new era*. Oxford: Oxford University Press; 2009. pp.63–83.

Logan S, Bedford H. Implementing immunization programmes. In: Lindstrom B, Spencer N, editors. *Social Paediatrics*. Oxford: Oxford University Press; 1995. pp.498–511.

McKee M. Public health in Central and Eastern Europe and the former Soviet Union. In: Beaglehole R, Bonita R, editors. *Global Public Health: a new era*. Oxford: Oxford University Press; 2009. pp.101–21.

Oliver TR. The politics of public health policy. *Annu Rev Public Health*. 2006; 27: 195–233.

Sharma M, Atri A. *Essentials of International Health*. Sudbury, MA: Jones and Bartlett; 2010.

Thakker P, Reddy KS. Public health in India. In: Beaglehole R, Bonita R, editors. *Global Public Health: a new era*. Oxford: Oxford University Press; 2009. pp.209–24.

Wall S, Persson G, Weinehall L. Public health in Sweden: facts, visions, and lessons. In: Beaglehole R, Bonita R, editors. *Global Public Health: a new era*. Oxford: Oxford University Press; 2009. pp.85–100.

CHAPTER 12

Evaluation: principles and practice

EVALUATION AND RELATED CONCEPTS

A few definitions may be helpful. *Evaluation* simply means 'to determine the value of' something. A more precise of elaboration of this is: 'The critical assessment, on as objective a basis as possible, of the degree to which entire services or their component parts ... fulfil stated goals' (St Leger, cited by Blair *et al* 2010).

Evaluation, audit and monitoring are conceptually related terms but have subtly different meanings. *Monitoring* differs (at least in theory) from both evaluation and audit in that it is a form of data collection and analysis that is sustained over a prolonged time period. It may be undertaken to assess the progress of a specified intervention or simply to assess an aspect of population health in the context of health protection or healthcare management. Monitoring is often synonymous with *surveillance* though the former term implies a more passive and less analytical process than the latter. Epidemiological *surveillance* may be defined as: 'the systematic collection, analysis and dissemination of health data for the planning, implementation and evaluation of public health programmes' (Thacker *et al* 1988).

The essential attribute of a successful surveillance system is that it should not merely be a mechanism for data collection and analysis but that it should be linked to action. There is no point in identifying an outbreak of, say, meningitis unless it triggers a specific and effective public health response to isolate the initial cases and prevent the spread of the disease throughout the population. Sometimes the response may simply comprise further investigation. Registries of cancer, congenital anomalies and other diseases frequently identify possible clusters or other unusual phenomena that turn out to be due to chance, misclassification or other sources of error. If the cluster is real, the public health system is obliged to try to identify the cause and remove it as rapidly as possible to protect the population from further harm.

While surveillance is extremely important, in the context of needs assessment and health protection, for assessing the health status of a population over time and in identifying environmental, infectious or other risks that may arise to threaten it, the remainder of the chapter will focus on the evaluation of interventions.

WHAT IS EVALUATION FOR?

Evaluation is a crucial component of evidence-based practice because it generates the evidence. It fulfils two quite distinct roles: to inform decision making about the selection of the most appropriate interventions, and to determine the extent to which an intervention, once implemented, has achieved its objectives. In the former role, the evidence is generated *a priori*, in the latter *post hoc*.

First, evaluation has a fundamental *prospective* role in informing public health activities at the point when practitioners have to decide which intervention or set of interventions are likely to benefit their target populations. In this case, the purpose of evaluation is to generate evidence of *efficacy* – or what works in carefully controlled research conditions – on which to plan and implement interventions. That evidence is as robust as the methodology used to create it. High-quality research will generate more reliable evidence than low-quality studies.

Second, evaluation is used as a *retrospective* means of finding out how well an intervention has worked in practice. As explained in the Introduction, the public health approach comprises three steps that roughly approximate to the clinical tasks of diagnosis, treatment and follow-up. The third and final 'follow-up' public health step involves evaluating (or auditing) the intervention to determine its *effectiveness*. The results are recycled back to the objectives of the intervention in a dynamic feedback loop. That is essential so that evaluation can inform the design or delivery of the intervention. Practitioners use the results of the evaluation to identify the strengths and weaknesses of the intervention. They can then decide whether to maintain the intervention in its current form or to modify it. In any event, the evaluation will be useful for disseminating a critical account of the experience to colleagues working in similar fields.

There is often great confusion about the purpose of an evaluation. The question that has to be answered at the outset is this: is the evaluation intended to generate new, generalisable knowledge about the efficacy of the intervention or programme, or is its purpose to assess the effectiveness of an intervention or programme in a particular time and place? If the answer is the former, then the evaluation is a type of research that is designed to generate new knowledge; if the latter, it is an audit of performance that is used for management purposes. The methodological approaches to these two types of investigation are very different.

Evaluating efficacy

In the first type of evaluation (assessment of efficacy), epidemiologists assess a novel intervention by means of a research method that compares a process or outcome with a predetermined objective or with a control group. This kind of evaluation is used to generate generalisable new knowledge about the intervention of interest. While the preferred method is the randomised controlled trial (RCT), it may be difficult or impossible to perform one for practical or ethical reasons. Alternative methodologies to the RCT should not be rejected out of hand as they may yield valuable if less reliable information about efficacy. These include historical (cross-over) controlled trials, non-randomised controlled trials, observational (before-and-after) studies, time-series analyses and case–control studies. Before-and-after studies are particularly popular. This type of evaluation, whereby a population (sometimes along with controls) is assessed prior to and following an intervention, is potentially highly problematic because it may prove difficult to attribute any changes observed over time to the intervention rather than to extraneous (confounding) factors.

Even when new knowledge is required, the 'gold standard' evaluational research method – the randomised controlled trial – may not be necessary. That is because the key requirement of *equipoise* may not exist. Equipoise means that the investigator is equally uncertain about the likely effectiveness of each arm of the proposed trial. If there is strong evidence from observational studies or even, on occasions, from anecdotal experience that an intervention is either highly effective or highly ineffective, a trial is not necessary and would be unethical. Historical examples of interventions that were not subjected to rigorous trials include the early use of penicillin to treat lobar pneumonia and the wearing of seatbelts to prevent injuries in car crashes.

Evaluating effectiveness

By contrast, the second type of evaluation (assessment of effectiveness), sometimes described as audit, seeks to assess the extent to which an intervention (that has already been implemented by a public health or other agency) meets predetermined standards – of performance or results or both – that are regarded as constituting good practice. The intervention has usually been selected on the presumption that it should work, based either on the best available research evidence (of efficacy) or past experience. The audit process is designed to determine whether the intervention actually does work in practice and, if it does not, to reveal the reasons for failure. Within large organisations or programmes, evaluation or audit is essentially a type of performance management that usually involves careful financial accounting. (This form of evaluation is sometimes described as an assessment of *efficiency*.)

A key feature of evaluation in public health is its systematic nature and its linkage to an established theoretical framework. One such framework is that proposed by Donabedian (2003) in which the achievements of the intervention or programme, in relation to its objectives, are assessed across the three dimensions of structure – process – outcome. What do these terms mean?

➤ *Structure* refers to fixed resources or elements and how they are organised.
➤ *Process* describes what is done, how much, and by whom.
➤ *Outcome* is the (usually) predetermined change or impact that is achieved.

All three are important in public health although the outcome indicators may be accorded a pre-eminent status. In practice, process measures may be more feasible to identify because of the long-term nature of many public health outcomes. At an early stage, the investigators have to decide whether to collect quantitative or qualitative data, or a combination of the two, on each of these three dimensions.

ECONOMIC EVALUATION

Money matters. All public health interventions require the allocation of resources, including funds, personnel, equipment and time. In large organisations, whether privately or publicly funded, all of these resources have a price tag and the expenditure has to be justified by attempting to answer a key question: is this investment of money yielding or likely to yield the desired outcomes? One means of doing this, beyond mere financial accounting or audit, is to undertake an economic evaluation.

Health economists employ several methods for evaluating interventions. Cost–benefit analysis (CBA) compares the investment in a programme or activity with its outcome (such as improved life expectancy), all in terms of monetary values that are time-adjusted (on the assumption that the value of money invested or saved changes over time). Cost–effectiveness analysis (CEA) compares alternative pathways to achieving the same objective. Cost–utility analysis (CUA) is a variant of cost–effectiveness analysis in which the ratio of the costs and benefits is calculated and expressed as money per benefit gained. Unlike cost–benefit analyses, the benefits of CUAs are not necessarily expressed in monetary terms and often include a quality of life dimension. Favoured outcome indicators in these types of analysis include quality-adjusted life-years (QALYs) and disability-adjusted life-years (DALYs) (*see* Chapter 2).

The process of attaching monetary values to the various components of the economic equation is controversial, particularly in the case of CBA. The figures may appear superficially precise but they are often based on estimates derived from surveys (of, for example, the public's 'willingness to pay' either to secure a promised benefit or to avoid a negative outcome). Some of the costs and benefits may be speculative or intangible (such as 'quality of life') and thus subject to vigorous debate. Critics of economic evaluation argue that the methods are unreliable – costs are commonly underestimated while benefits are overestimated – or even unethical, since any attempt to apply monetary values to health, disability and death trivialises human suffering.

EVALUATION IN THE PLANNING CYCLE

Evaluation plays a key role in the public health planning cycle. It poses a series of inter-related questions: what are the objectives of the programme, service or policy? How are they being met? What are the results? What are the implications of the results for the programme, service or policy? If evaluation is undertaken, it should be linked – like audit – via feedback loops into the earlier stages of the planning cycle.

The timing of evaluation is crucial. While all interventions should be evaluated, a decision must be taken at an early stage whether to perform a formative or summative evaluation. A *formative evaluation* is undertaken during the development of a programme, enabling changes to be made in either the objectives or its implementation. This type of evaluation is embedded within the delivery of the intervention. It frequently focuses on staff or participant attitudes, performance or satisfaction. By contrast, a *summative evaluation* usually comes later in the process and is designed to offer insights into the effectiveness of a programme over a defined period of time. Summative evaluation is helpful to planners in deciding whether to continue, expand, modify or terminate an established programme

Dahlberg and Stone (Box 12.1) indicated how public health professionals with responsibility for violence prevention might set about an evaluation in the context of planning and implementing an intervention programme. They outlined five interlinked steps: clarify the programme goals or objectives, design an evaluation plan, develop and implement a data collection plan, analyse and interpret the data, and use and report the findings. The process is a sequential and cyclical one (Fig. 12.1).

The cyclical model emphasises the interconnections between the various steps. Having a clear idea of the programme's goals and objectives is obviously a prerequisite of the entire evaluation. Outcome evaluation is especially challenging and should never be conducted in isolation. It is especially important that outcomes are judged in the context of both the objectives and the process; all of this information is essential to understanding whether or not the programme worked, and in revealing precisely what went right or what went wrong.

THE SPECIAL CASE OF SCREENING

These general principles of evaluation are widely applicable. There are, however, a few circumstances in which special evaluation principles or criteria have been developed. A particularly relevant one for public health is screening or

---

BOX 12.1 *Evaluation of public health interventions: guidelines for professionals using the five-step evaluation model**

Step 1: clarify programme goals/objectives
What is a goal? It is a general statement about what you are trying to achieve. Objectives indicate how the goal will be achieved. NB: Objectives should be SMART – specific, measurable, action-oriented, realistic and time-specific.

Step 2: design an evaluation plan
➤ Decide who is your target audience.
➤ Clarify time scale and resources.
➤ Select an evaluation framework (e.g. structure – process – outcome).
➤ Choose an appropriate evaluation method.

Step 3: develop and implement a data collection plan
➤ Decide whether to collect *quantitative* or *qualitative* data – or both.
➤ Choose specific types of data to collect (e.g. demographic, mortality, self-report, observational).
➤ Collect the data.

Step 4: analyse and interpret the data
➤ Prepare the data for analysis.
➤ Analyse the data.
➤ Interpret the results.

Step 5: use and report your findings
➤ Select your audience (e.g. policy, academic) depending on purpose.
➤ Present findings in appropriate format.
➤ Recommend, where necessary, changes to the programme.

*Based on Dahlberg L, Stone D. Workshop on Outcome Evaluation. WHO Third Milestones of a Global Campaign of Violence Prevention, Scotland, 2007.

---

early detection of disease through mass testing of a population. Screening has become one of the key preventive strategies of public health since the mid-20th century and is often mired in controversy.

The UK National Screening Committee (2010) defines screening as follows:

> Screening is a process of identifying apparently healthy people who may be at increased risk of a disease or condition. They can then be offered information, further tests and appropriate treatment to reduce their risk and/or any complications arising from the disease or condition.

Five step evaluation model

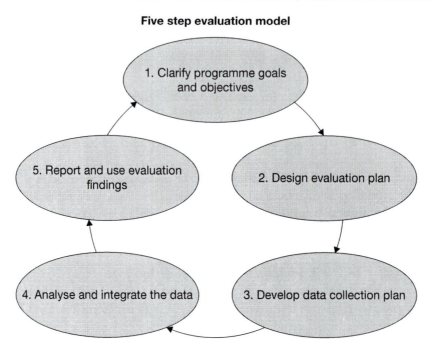

Figure 12.1 A cyclical approach to evaluation. Source: Dahlberg L, Stone D. Workshop on Outcome Evaluation. WHO Third Milestones of a Global Campaign of Violence Prevention, Scotland, 2007.

Screening may be advocated for the early identification and avoidance of risk factors (e.g. alcohol misuse, smoking), for the early detection of signs of disease (e.g. postnatal depression) that require specific clinical or social interventions, and for the early diagnosis of important and potentially debilitating sequelae of disease or injury (e.g. post-traumatic stress disorder). Based on the apparently impeccable logic that early diagnosis will ensure better prognosis, screening is an idea that is enormously appealing to professionals and the public alike. Rather than wait for a disease to reach such an advanced stage that any form of treatment becomes futile, identifying symptoms and signs at an earlier stage is bound to offer a much better prospect of cure. In practice, that premise turns out to be dubious: not only does screening often fail to improve prognosis, it may actually be counterproductive by generating anxiety, additional work and expense, and producing side-effects and complications of unnecessary diagnostic or therapeutic procedures. In some cases, screening merely results in a longer period of known disease.

Screening poses uniquely awkward ethical problems for public health planners. Unusually in healthcare, it is a form of clinical intervention that is anticipatory rather than responsive. In conventional clinical care, a patient with a symptom or a problem approaches the health service for advice and, where

appropriate, diagnostic procedures are undertaken followed, if thought necessary, by treatment. The healthcare professional responds to the patient's pre-
sentation with no prior promise of success. Screening, by contrast, is offered
to people who have not usually sought help. In other words, it is undertaken
at the initiative of the service rather than the patient. The implication is that
screening will confer some benefit, otherwise it would not be offered to the
public. That obliges those who offer screening to the public to be reasonably
confident, in advance, that the programme will ultimately benefit at least some
of those screened. If that confidence is absent or misplaced, the screening programme should not be implemented.

After the Second World War, the development of mass diagnostic technologies such as portable radiography and laboratory auto-analysers resulted in a
rapid proliferation of screening programmes in several industrialised countries.
Healthcare providers, governments and clinicians, who came under increasing pressure from commercial organisations and the media to exploit the new
technologies, urgently sought guidance on the introduction of screening programmes. At the request of the WHO, Wilson and Jungner (1968) laid out a
set of principles that drew attention to the need to consider carefully the pros
and cons of screening prior to the implementation of a programme. These have
stood the test of time well. The special characteristics of screening have led to
the formulation of principles or criteria for the purposes either of considering
whether or not to implement a screening programme, or to evaluate an established one, or both. These criteria may be grouped under three headings: ethical, scientific and economic.

The *ethical* criteria include: a demonstration that the problem is an important one from a public health perspective; the screening test should reach the
population at risk; the screening test must be acceptable to the subjects; effective treatment should be available should screening reveal a disorder; and the
benefits of screening should be known to outweigh the harm. The *scientific*
criteria include: the natural history (including the preclinical time span) of
the disorder should be understood; the validity of the screening test, or its
ability to separate the screened population into those who have this disorder (sensitivity) from those who do not (specificity), should be known; and
a clear consensus on what constitutes a positive test result should exist. The
economic criteria include: an understanding of the resource requirements of
screening and the subsequent investigations and follow-up; the economic costs
and benefits should be known with the latter outweighing the former; and the
opportunity costs (i.e. the costs of diverting resources away from other activities towards screening) should be estimated.

Underpinning all these principles is a common theme: public health professionals should be prepared to challenge the widespread assumption, often
based on inadequate evidence, that earlier detection of a disorder or risk fac-

tor through screening is always beneficial to the population that is screened. Although there are several examples of highly successful screening programmes (e.g. for neonatal disorders such as hypothyroidism or for coronary heart disease risk factors in middle-aged adults), the reality is that the claims made on behalf of screening are often unjustified or wildly exaggerated. All public health practitioners and policy makers should be constantly alert to the widely underestimated pitfalls of screening.

CONCLUDING REFLECTIONS ON EVALUATION

The gap between the theory and practice of evaluation may be wide. Being aware of some of the most common practical pitfalls confronting practitioners and policy makers should help in their avoidance. The most important principle of evaluation is that it obliges practitioners to ask the fundamental question: does this intervention work? Good intentions are insufficient. And a subsidiary question that a robust evaluation should answer is almost equally important: are there any negative effects of the intervention? In the research context, RCTs are notoriously poor at detecting adverse effects unless these are carefully incorporated into the study design. And service evaluators always need to be alert to negative as well as positive outcomes. Even if an intervention is shown to be neutral in its impact – neither positive nor negative – that finding is valuable as it prompts questions about the opportunity cost (the diversion of resources away from other potentially valuable interventions).

Performing research of the requisite quality is a major challenge for the public health community because of the complexity, scale and expense of many of the interventions of interest. Few shortcuts are available to evaluational researchers and attempts to find them often lead to heated disputes between purists and pragmatists, with the former arguing for RCTs (the gold standard of evaluation) as the methodology of first choice and the latter willing to adopt less rigorous approaches for pragmatic reasons. Readers will decide for themselves where they feel comfortable along this spectrum of opinion. The essential point is that there are no absolutes in the realms of either evaluational research or the interpretation of the evidence that it yields. Some specialists (Greenhalgh 1997) in critical appraisal and evidence-based medicine have proposed a 'hierarchy of evidence' with systematic reviews and meta-analyses (in which the results of individual trials are pooled) at the top of the hierarchy and case reports at the bottom (*see* Chapter 8).

Feelings can run surprisingly high about evaluation, perhaps because value judgements are inevitably involved. There is often a gulf of understanding between researchers and practitioners. The latter may regard evaluation as 'academic theory' with little practical relevance, or even a potential threat to their professional integrity or competence. Many public health practitioners have spent their careers participating in activities that have not been evaluated and they may feel vulnerable when exposed to the implications of an evaluation's findings. Others may be stubbornly resistant to the notion that some interventions, long entrenched and believed to be worthwhile, may turn out to be wholly or partially ineffective. The excessive and sustained attachment of some practitioners to health education as a linchpin of health promotion, despite the largely disappointing body of research evidence on its efficacy, is an illustration of this phenomenon.

The results of an evaluation may be unsatisfactory or contentious for methodological reasons, such as a low statistical power arising from too small a sample size. If an evaluation suggests a lack of effectiveness, practitioners may challenge the results on the basis of allegedly inappropriate methodology rather than any inherent deficiencies in the intervention or in its implementation. The selection and measurement of outcome indicators may be particularly contentious. For that reason, the methodological approach to evaluation should be agreed in advance with stakeholders who should then be asked to commit themselves to respecting the findings. While the main focus of the evaluation may be on outcomes, process indicators should not be overlooked. If implementation is inadequate or flawed, the desired outcomes cannot be achieved.

Evaluation may be performed internally by programme staff or externally by independent investigators. The former is more practical while the latter is more objective. Ideally, a combination of both is used. Internal evaluation should be an integral part of implementation. But restricting evaluation to an internal exercise, in which the participants may be perceived as having a vested interest, risks seriously damaging the credibility of the whole programme. Evaluation should not only be conducted impartially and objectively, it should be transparent in its methodology and free of conflicting or compromising pressures.

Evaluation is sometimes dismissed as a dry, academic pursuit. In reality, it tends to be a pragmatic, practical, problem-oriented and creative activity. It can also be highly divisive because so much is at stake when an evaluation is conducted. As well as providing insights into whether or not a specific intervention has achieved its objectives, evaluation studies may be used to judge the effectiveness and efficiency of entire organisations, departments and programmes. Evaluation is an activity that can make or break reputations and careers, generate or destroy jobs, and unlock or freeze scarce resources. In short, evaluation is of such paramount importance to public health, and so potentially controversial, that no public health practitioner or policy maker can afford to neglect it.

REFERENCES

Blair M, Stewart-Brown S, Waterston T, *et al. Child Public Health.* 2nd ed. Oxford: Oxford University Press; 2010.

Donabedian A. *An Introduction to Quality Assurance in Health Care*. New York: Oxford University Press; 2003.

Greenhalgh T. Getting your bearings (deciding what the paper is about). *BMJ*. 1997; **315**: 243–6.

Thacker SB, Parrish RG, Trowbridge FL. A method for evaluating systems of epidemiological surveillance. *World Health Stat Q*. 1988; **41**: 11–18.

UK National Screening Committee. *UK Screening Portal. Programme appraisal criteria*. 2010. www.screening.nhs.uk/criteria

Wilson JMG, Jungner G. *Principles and Practice of Screening for Disease*. Geneva: World Health Organization; 1968.

CHAPTER 13

The quest for new knowledge

EVIDENCE-BASED PUBLIC HEALTH DEPENDS ON KNOWLEDGE

Modern public health is a science-based discipline. Without science and technology, much of the improvement in global health over the last century would have been impossible. We would have lacked many of the products, devices, drugs and procedures we take for granted, such as diagnostic tests, vaccines, drugs, intravenous lines, endoscopes, and a huge range of therapeutic and operative equipment. We would have known little about the nature and importance to human health of bacteria, viruses, parasites and other pathogenic micro-organisms, and how to confront them. We would have remained blissfully ignorant of the causes and risk factors for disease, genetics, health hazards and methods of environmental conservation. And we would have been unable to undertake rigorous epidemiological research, including randomised controlled trials of novel therapies, or to mount nutritional, screening or family planning programmes, or to develop other evidence-based strategies for health improvement.

Generating new knowledge is the *raison d'être* of researchers and academics. That knowledge is essential to the public health tasks of assessing needs, elucidating causes, implementing effective interventions and evaluating their impact. At one time, many healthcare professionals viewed research as an intellectual, almost esoteric, pursuit with minimal relevance to the real world. All of that has changed with the growing recognition of the need to base key decisions on good-quality evidence. Without recourse to a steady stream of high-quality research outputs disseminated through peer-reviewed publications, public health professionals will struggle to practise evidence-based public health.

The sources of new knowledge on public health are rapidly multiplying thanks to the growing number of active researchers around the world combined with spectacular developments in information technology, particularly the internet. This phenomenal growth in the availability of scientific information, while welcome, is a double-edged sword. It is indisputable that public health practitioners have access to more high-quality research data than at any time in history. At the same time, the sheer volume of new information is impossible to assimilate and update in the course of daily work. That challenge has, in turn, spawned a new kind of professional – the specialist in critical appraisal, translational research and knowledge transfer.

WHAT NEW KNOWLEDGE DO WE NEED?

Epidemiology and related disciplines are powerful tools for investigating the causes and courses (natural histories) of disease. Traditional case–control and cohort studies remain useful for these purposes but methodological innovation has been slow. And many epidemiologists have been reluctant to extend these approaches beyond the investigation of risk factors for chronic disease in affluent countries to the study of other types of disorders in the world as a whole. Broader or 'macro' social, environmental, cultural, economic and political influences on health are now widely recognised but rarely subjected to rigorous scientific scrutiny. At a global level, the effects of the demographic and epidemiological transitions, conflict, terrorism, climate change, environmental disruption and migration on health and wellbeing deserve far greater attention from public health researchers. At the same time, the scope for deepening understanding of specific diseases, particularly those that continue to devastate large areas of the globe, remains vast.

Epidemiology began as the systematic investigation of epidemics of communicable diseases. That role has never been rendered redundant. As well as the 'big three' infectious killers (TB, HIV/AIDS and malaria) that continue to devastate individual lives, families, communities and countries, millions of people still fall victim annually to microbe-induced diarrhoeal diseases, respiratory disorders, parasitic infections and other forms of sepsis. Epidemiologists try to describe and quantify the toll of suffering incurred by all of these diseases as well as mortality and morbidity arising from non-infectious causes such as malnutrition, vitamin deficiencies, diabetes, cancer, cardiovascular disease and mental illness. A group of so-called 'neglected diseases' account for around a quarter of the annual DALYs from communicable diseases and demand a renewed research effort. These include helminthic infections such as hookworm, lymphatic filariasis (elephantiasis), onchocerciasis (river blindness), schistosomiasis and dracunculiasis (guinea worm), protozoal infections such as leishmaniasis (kal-azar), trypanosomiasis (sleeping sickness and Chagas' disease), and bacterial infections such as trachoma and leprosy.

The Global Burden of Disease study (*see* Chapter 2) demonstrated the utility of descriptive epidemiology, and the value of new population health indicators such as QALYs and DALYs that combine mortality and disability, in making a public health diagnosis. Further methodological development of this and similar approaches is needed, and is currently under way, to maximise its potential. We still know far too little about the total numbers of deaths, their causes and their potential avoidability. Even larger gaps exist in our knowledge of disease incidence, case fatality, disability, psychological wellbeing and quality of life. Disease registers and *ad hoc* surveys are often difficult to organise and too expensive to meet the needs of poorer countries so alternative approaches have to be explored.

Probably the single most pressing question facing global public health today is how to improve health without reinforcing or widening inequalities. Although we are gaining an increasingly sophisticated understanding of how inequalities in health are produced, our knowledge of how to reverse them remains patchy. Many well-intentioned national and international public health and social policies seem to have made little or no impact on this intractable problem. Why is this? Morgan and Ziglio (2007) offer four explanations. First, the underlying causes of health inequalities are numerous, complex, intergenerational and interacting. Researchers have barely scratched the surface of the subject, either in terms of their nature or their detailed causal pathways. Much more large-scale, adequately funded, long-term epidemiological and aetiological research is required. Second, even when disease aetiology is reasonably well understood, empirical evidence of the efficacy of interventions in narrowing health inequalities is inadequate. Third, the translation of research-based evidence of efficacy into effective action in the field often falls short of expectations, partly because of the neglect of the various factors that facilitate or obstruct implementation. Finally, the authors believe that too much research has focused on the 'deficit model' (identification of problems or failures) or health and disease rather than the 'asset model' (identification of resilience and solutions). They call for a reorientation of public health research on the reinforcement of assets rather than the countering of deficits, in line with the salutogenic (health-promoting) theories of Antonovsky (1979).

Since poverty plays such a prominent role in the aetiology of so many diseases, more effective poverty reduction measures would pay public health dividends. Within countries, fiscal and welfare policies designed to boost economic growth and redistribute wealth appear the most promising strategies to reduce relative poverty. Globally, economic stagnation is the biggest obstacle to growth in the poorest countries. To help boost economic growth in affected regions, Sachs (2005) suggests six areas deserving of special attention from the international research community:

➤ preventive, diagnostic and therapeutic measures for diseases prevalent in low-income countries
➤ tropical agricultural techniques such as the development of new seed varieties and soil management
➤ energy systems for remote rural areas that require off-grid power from renewable sources

➤ climate forecasting over longer time spans, enabling better prediction of and adjustment to severe weather events
➤ water management, including desalination, irrigation and water conservation
➤ sustainable management of fragile ecosystems such as coral reefs, mangrove swamps, fisheries and rainforests.

A particularly pressing topic for further research is climate change. Poor countries are likely to suffer disproportionately from rising ocean levels, changing patterns of rainfall and temperature variation, the toxic effects of carbon dioxide and other climate shocks. A greater investment in climate science and related disciplines is necessary to enable all countries, but especially the developing countries, to respond effectively to these major challenges to economic prosperity and health.

THE UNTAPPED POTENTIAL OF SCIENCE AND TECHNOLOGY

Addressing the mismatch between scientific and technological advances and their effective application (the implementation gap) is a perennial challenge for public health and is a legitimate, important and neglected subject for research. Skolnik (2008) reminds us of the huge health gains that could be achieved globally were existing knowledge and technologies (many of which are low cost) fully implemented. He cites six examples of measures that are known to be efficacious but are currently insufficiently applied.

➤ Better hygiene practices, including hand washing.
➤ Promoting exclusive breastfeeding for six months.
➤ Expanding coverage of the population with the six basic vaccines (against diphtheria, tetanus, pertussis, polio, tuberculosis and measles) to reduce infant infection rates.
➤ Increasing case finding and cure rates of TB by using the DOTS (Directly Observed Therapy, Short-course) approach.
➤ Improved diagnosis of obstetric complications along with speedy transport to hospital for emergency care.
➤ Enhancing birth attendants' skills in neonatal resuscitation, provision of antibiotics and keeping babies warm.

There are many other opportunities for narrowing the implementation gap: reducing the costs of AIDS drugs to increase the proportion of sufferers treated, distributing more widely insecticide-treated bed nets to improve malaria control, expanding family planning services, ensuring the universal availability of oral rehydration solutions for the treatment of diarrhoea, and the strengthening of the effectiveness and efficiency of healthcare systems.

Harnessing the potential of science and technology to the demands of global public health has the potential to secure further breakthroughs in the future. Around the start of the millennium, a panel of 28 experts was invited to identify ways in which biotechnology could help to improve health in developing countries within the next decade (Daar *et al* 2002). They concluded that the top priorities for development were diagnostic techniques, vaccines and drugs, in that order, followed by water purification, sanitation and products that would empower women to protect themselves against sexually transmitted diseases. If that panel were reconvened today, it would hardly be surprising if their list of priorities remained much the same, perhaps with the addition of two topics they may have overlooked: the implications of the Human Genome Project for the identification, prevention and treatment of disease and risk factors; and the role of information technology for health education, practitioner skill development, individual and community empowerment, and public participation in policy making and evaluation.

In 2003, the Bill and Melinda Gates Foundation, in conjunction with several international partner organisations, launched an ambitious programme of research designed to confront global health problems. The Grand Challenges in Global Health scheme has supported efforts to improve existing childhood vaccines, develop new vaccines and drugs, improve vaccine transport and delivery systems, control disease-transmitting insects such as mosquitoes, improve nutrition and cure chronic infection. Initiatives such as this are crucial as advances in the development of vaccines, drugs, devices and other products are unlikely to emerge from either the public sector, that tends to be risk averse, or private industry, that sees little prospect of a profitable return on investment. Skolnik (2008) proposes a dual strategy for overcoming market failure by deploying a combination of 'push' and 'pull' mechanisms. The former would lower the cost of research and development for the private sector through government financing and tax credits. The latter would ensure a satisfactory return on investment through government subsidies and incentives at the point when the product is available.

TRANSLATIONAL RESEARCH FOR PUBLIC HEALTH

The ultimate purpose of epidemiology is to inform public health policy making and practice. Knowledge transfer between epidemiological researchers and public health service providers is necessary to ensure that the latter make evidence-based decisions. The need for translational research is as paramount within public health as it is within clinical disciplines though this is not always acknowledged explicitly. The literature contains few examples of the successful deployment of translational research in public health. The gap between academia and public health practitioners is real and may be traced to several causes, notably divergent aims (generating new knowledge versus service delivery) and the practical obstacles to routine collaborative working. The formalisation of knowledge transfer and exchange within the field of public health policy is still at an early stage. A systematic review on the use of research evidence by health policy makers (Innvær *et al* 2002) used interviews and surveys with key health policy decision makers to gain a better understanding of the barriers to the application of research evidence. From the 24 studies from around the world that met their inclusion criteria, they concluded that two-way communication between researcher and policy maker was essential. They also warned against the selective use, whether inadvertent or deliberate, of evidence by policy makers.

Beaglehole and Bonita (1997) attribute some of the implementation gap between evidence and policy to the allegedly malign role of vested interests such as manufacturers of dangerous substances. In support of this view, they cite the continuing inaction to prevent the spread of the tobacco epidemic throughout the world despite the overwhelming evidence of the harmful effects of smoking on health. At the same time, they take many members of the research community to task for maintaining a professional distance from their scientific and policy colleagues, and from the general public, in an effort to maintain scientific purity. Too many epidemiologists seem to enjoy working in splendid isolation and seem either unaware of or indifferent to the complexities and multifaceted demands of policy making.

PUBLIC HEALTH IS UNDERPINNED BY CHANGING SCIENTIFIC PARADIGMS

Public health has evolved in many ways, not least in its attachment to successive scientific theories or paradigms. These paradigms are important as they can determine the direction of research and practice for decades. In its early period, the miasma theory of disease was dominant but this gave way to an environmental one as the role of unsanitary and overcrowded living conditions in promoting epidemics was recognised in the 18th and early 19th centuries. The environmental paradigm, in turn, gave way to the microbiological one following the discovery of bacteria and other micro-organisms in the late 19th century. Bacteriology dominated public health until the mid-20th century when social welfare reform was believed to hold the key to better health. By the end of that century, the individual risk factor approach, focusing largely on lifestyle and behaviour, seemed to offer the best prospects for health improvement.

By the start of the 21st century, the explosion of genetic knowledge offered yet another paradigm whereby disease would be predicted and conquered by molecular biology and genetic engineering. That is competing with alternative models that place greater emphasis on a whole raft of new or rediscovered theories and value systems. Among these are clinical interventions designed to improve health (such as screening and anticipatory healthcare), econometrics (boosted by financial austerity), ecological and environmental justice perspectives, human rights and social justice advocacy, programming (whether biological, psychological or social) across the life cycle (*see* Chapter 4), intergenerational epidemiology and epigenetics, and information technology. Today, we may be witnessing an intriguing phenomenon whereby many of the older paradigms are being integrated into a new, complex and over-arching holistic theory of health that attempts to take account of biological, familial, social, environmental, economic and cultural influences that interact with each other across the lifecourse to cause disease or improve health. A core feature of this embryonic new paradigm will presumably be an emphasis on the inter-relationships (often unrecognised) between the various non-health professionals, agencies and departments that have an indirect remit for health and wellbeing. These include, among many others, sectors that deal with education, social services, justice, transport, migration, product safety, economic productivity, food, agriculture, water management, energy, climate, biodiversity and the environment in its broadest sense.

As in other branches of science, epidemiological findings are often misunderstood or misreported by the media. One way in which epidemiologists and other public health researchers can influence policy and practice to a greater degree is to improve their methods of measuring and communicating risk. Relative risks, for example, are generally higher and more impressive than population-attributable risks. While the former tend to be favoured by epidemiologists in scientific papers, the latter are actually more relevant to public health. Moreover, the application of batteries of statistical tests to determine the 'significance' of relative risks is liable to generate many spurious associations that are the result of artefact, bias, chance, misclassification, unrecognised (confounding) variables or other sources of error rather than real and biologically plausible phenomena. Beaglehole and Bonita (1997) suggest that many of these failings may be traced to the tendency of epidemiologists to remain wedded to a narrow and outmoded scientific paradigm that they characterise as 'biomedical individualism'. The result is an excessive focus on personal risk factors rather than social, environmental or cultural ones and an overinterpretation of statistically significant associations.

CONCLUDING THOUGHTS ABOUT PUBLIC HEALTH RESEARCH

Public health research may be either fundamental (mainly epidemiology) or applied (or goal oriented). Both may be subsumed under the generic heading of 'research and development' and both have key roles to play in knowledge generation to inform global public health decision making and improve its effectiveness. The global public health research effort spans a huge field, embracing epidemiology, healthcare research, biostatistics, health metrics, health economics, and the wider social sciences as well as related clinical, laboratory and information technology fields.

Like most research, public health research is time consuming, labour intensive, difficult and (sometimes) expensive. But it labours under several additional burdens that do not afflict other forms of research to the same extent. First and foremost of these is its lack of critical mass. Although public health research has been expanding in recent decades, both in volume and scope, it remains insufficient to meet the enormous scale and complexity of the challenge. There are numerous, interconnected reasons for this.

First, research skills remain too scarce in the public health field to meet the needs of the specialty. All countries and regions suffer from weak capacity for public health research (especially for the investigation of global health) due to an absence of training, career structures and job security in academic or other settings where research is pursued. Poorer countries are especially vulnerable to the globalised market in public health skills as trained practitioners often experience frustration and minimal prospects for career advancement in their home countries. The resultant 'brain drain' to the richer world is well documented and extremely damaging to the exporting countries.

Second, there are too many investigators chasing too little money. Laboratory and clinical research departments tend to be much more generously funded than epidemiology units. That is partly a reflection of the paucity of trained researchers with the necessary skills to raise grants and conduct research. But we also need to overcome the problems associated with what might be described as the superficially unglamorous nature of much public research. Somehow this negative image must be overturned as it is responsible, in large part, for the relatively miserly resource allocation to public health research programmes in the face of competition from apparently more deserving causes.

Third, funding bodies are sometimes sceptical of the utility of much public health research. This resistance is a legacy of the past when public health research was less sophisticated, and may change as the evidence-based movement ensures that more effort than ever before is invested in synthesising the results of the research conducted by epidemiologists. A further problem is the gap between knowledge and its implementation. Organisations such as the Cochrane Collaboration have contributed enormously to the development of critical appraisal skills and to the dissemination of the findings of research in a way that is useful to practitioners. And yet many of the insights achieved through systematic reviews, meta-analyses and practice guidelines have not been properly translated into public health action. That may be due, in turn, to our failure to use research methods more consistently to identify and overcome the obstacles to the application of existing knowledge. More implementation research is needed to investigate the reasons for this.

Finally, the global public health research effort is unfocused and unco-ordinated. Strategic thinking in public health research is extremely rare. The current *ad hoc*, arbitrary and unplanned manner in which most public health research is conducted is inefficient and unlikely to achieve optimal impact. Researchers and international stakeholders (notably the WHO) need to work together more productively to develop a global public health research strategy that is designed to meet the information needs of policy makers and practitioners in the 21st century.

REFERENCES

Antonovsky A. *Health, Stress and Coping*. San Francisco: Jossey-Bass; 1979.

Beaglehole R, Bonita R. *Public Health at the Crossroads: achievements and prospects*. Cambridge: Cambridge University Press; 1997.

Daar AS, Thorsteindottir H, Martin DK, *et al*. Top ten biotechnologies for improving health in developing countries. *Nat Genet*. 2002; **32**: 229–32.

Innvær S, Vist G, Trommald M, *et al*. Health policy-makers' perceptions of their use of evidence: a systematic review. *J Health Serv Res Policy*. 2002; **7**(4): 239–44.

Morgan A, Ziglio E. Revitalising the evidence base for public health: the assets model. *Promot Educ Suppl*. 2007; **2**: 17–22.

Sachs J. *The End of Poverty*. London: Penguin Books; 2005.

Skolnik R. *Essentials of Global Health*. Sudbury, MA: Jones and Bartlett Learning; 2008.

CHAPTER 14

Holding the public health community to account

ETHICAL AND LEGAL ASPECTS OF PUBLIC HEALTH POLICY AND PRACTICE

Ethics of epidemiological research

As epidemiology is the basic science of public health, it is germane to consider its ethical dimensions here. In common with other biomedical researchers, epidemiologists are bound, at least in principle, by the Helsinki Declaration that requires that research with humans should conform to accepted scientific principles, and should be truthful, honest, impartial and objective. Originally based on the Nuremberg Code of 1947 (articulated in response to the discovery of brutal Nazi medical experimentation during the Second World War), the Declaration has undergone six revisions and two clarifications since its first version was published in 1964. Its key principle relates to informed consent, particularly when research subjects are vulnerable to exploitation. Other principles cover the welfare of the participants, the avoidance of conflicts of interest and related aspects of publication ethics, and the use of placebos in clinical trials.

The main operational principles arising from the Helsinki Declaration state that research should:

➤ be based on a thorough knowledge of the scientific background (Article 11)
➤ take account of a careful assessment of risks and benefits (Articles 16, 17)
➤ have a reasonable likelihood of benefit to the population studied (Article 19)
➤ be conducted by suitably trained investigators (Article 15) using approved protocols, subject to independent ethical review and oversight by a properly convened committee (Article 13)
➤ be based on a protocol that is in compliance with the Declaration (Article 14).

The Helsinki Declaration may appear at first sight to be relevant only to exper-imental biological or clinical research on human subjects but it also covers research involving identifiable data derived from human participants. Even where epidemiologists use non-identifiable data, ethical principles are appli-cable. A frequent difficulty is the conflict between the protection of personal privacy and the use of health and other records for epidemiological research. Large-scale studies employing linked databases pose particular challenges. Many jurisdictions around the world have been grappling with this dilemma with only partial success.

Epidemiologists face many other ethical quandaries. Research funded by the pharmaceutical, tobacco or alcohol industries may prompt suspicion of conflict of interests to the point where any findings become unpublishable in respected scientific journals. Paying incentives, expenses or other rewards to study participants may be judged, in some circumstances, to amount to exploitation of vulnerable people. Performing research, including randomised controlled trials, in poor communities or countries may also raise questions about possible exploitation, inadequate explanation or failure to benefit the participants. And the extent to which researchers should become advocates for specific public health interventions is controversial since their impartiality and objectivity may appear to be compromised.

The specific role of ethics committees as watchdogs of behavioural stan-dards within the research community is controversial. In many countries, the approval of an ethical committee is mandatory before a study can proceed. This seems a reasonable means of preventing fraud or other forms of malpractice, for controlling commercial or governmental exploitation of participants and data, and for the protection of human subjects from harm, intentional or inad-vertent. Few would argue against these laudable aims. In practice, while the ethical oversight of research seems to work fairly well in most cases, there are egregious instances where unethically conducted research has slipped through the net. A notorious study that appeared to show a link between a vaccine and autism achieved publication in the respected British medical journal *The Lan-cet* in 1998 despite several layers of ethical safeguards, all of which failed. The paper was subsequently retracted by the journal.

Epidemiologists are equally concerned about the opposite phenomenon whereby ethics committees obstruct the performance of high-quality research for apparently arbitrary or capricious, if well-meaning, reasons. In some cases, excessive concern about the risk of a proposed study breaching legislation on data confidentiality, privacy and consent may prompt an ethical objection. In others, a misunderstanding of the important role of controls in the design of RCTs may endanger ethical approval. Ethics committees rarely contemplate the negative effects their zealotry may have on scientific progress and hence public health improvement. The prolixity of the debate surrounding the aetiological role of folate deficiency in neural tube defects may be attributed, in large part, to the initial reluctance of an ethics committee to approve the undertaking of RCTs of folate supplementation that would have established its efficacy much earlier (Scott *et al* 1994).

Ethics of public health practice

> Public health ... is arguably the health field most affected by human rights realities and by governmental successes or failures to respect, protect, and fulfil those rights. (Beyrer 2007)

The principles of ethical professional behaviour and practice have now been well established in relation to clinical disciplines. These need to be extended to public health practice in all its forms. Reference has already been made to the centrality of the human rights approach to health, and vice versa, at least since the Second World War. Health and human rights are widely regarded as mutually reinforcing. Moreover, one cannot be denied without affecting the other. That logic has been integral to the various international declarations on both human rights and health.

Public health has always been concerned with equity (including universal access to healthcare and other services), fairness and social justice, though there are divergent views within its ranks as to how these ethical values should be interpreted. The perennial issue of health inequalities is now regarded as central to the public health endeavour and has even been included in some definitions of public health (*see* Introduction). A variant of this concern is the focus on marginal and vulnerable groups such as children, women, the elderly and the disabled as well as the particular health needs of ethnic, religious and sexual minorities. And some scenarios, such as responding to the HIV/AIDS pandemic or dealing with humanitarian disasters, pose peculiarly acute ethical dilemmas due to their scale, urgency or contentious moral or political undercurrents.

The healthcare and related professions cannot function in the absence of trust. The general public – potential patients and clients – must have confidence in these professions to enable care (and prevention) to be delivered effectively. Although trust is an intangible asset, its preservation is vital and depends on the ability of professionals to demonstrate to the public a commitment to high standards of competence and behaviour. That commitment is demonstrable via a collective adherence to a set of moral principles that are either implicit or explicitly enshrined in codes of professional practice. Professional bodies such as the UK General Medical Council and the medical Royal Colleges (including the multidisciplinary Faculty of Public Health) promulgate and uphold these codes through their responsibility, often backed by statute, to monitor and maintain professional standards.

Ethics refers to the rules or standards governing the conduct of a person or the members of a profession. Those standards are underpinned by implicit or explicit moral values. Drawing on the work of American ethicists, Gillon (1994) argued that healthcare workers should be guided by four fundamental *prima facie* moral principles:

➤ autonomy (respect for individual rights)
➤ beneficence (doing good)
➤ non-maleficence (avoiding doing harm)
➤ justice (ensuring fairness)

along with a concern for the context in which the principles are applied.

Gillon's four principles, though not immune to criticism, have won broad acceptance among clinicians. They are simple, logical and culturally neutral. They are also easily understood by the intelligent lay observer. Nevertheless, problems may arise when they are applied, in unmodified form, to public health.

A commonly expressed reservation about the application of healthcare ethics to public health is that the codes were developed in the context of the care of individuals rather than populations. At first sight, this seems a churlish objection. After all, populations comprise individuals and the four principles seem perfectly capable of being applied to large numbers of individuals ('a population') in a manner that does not differ fundamentally from the approach of clinicians. To put it another way, while the scope of application of the principles is larger in scale in public health than in clinical practice, the principles themselves are equally relevant. That view, while superficially appealing, is now recognised as inadequate. The ethics of public health are quite distinct from those of clinical practice in many respects.

While clinical medicine and some other healthcare fields have developed ethical codes of practice that relate to the interaction between professionals and individuals in ways that fulfil Gillon's four key moral principles, public health workers face an entirely different, or at least far more complex, set of moral imperatives (Wikler and Cash 2009). These include advocating a fairer distribution of resources and promoting interventions that are designed to create a more socially equitable society. Both of these demand an awareness of the role of collective interests and responsibilities, and the dilemmas inherent in commitments and actions to promote and protect the health of groups, communities and populations. To complicate matters further, the particular ethical conundrums posed by disease prevention and the healthcare provision to vulnerable groups, such as young children, the elderly or the disabled, become even more challenging when scaled up to population-level public health practice and policy making.

Conflicts may arise between the rights of communities to be protected from health hazards on the one hand and those of some individuals to pursue their own chosen lifestyles on the other. Three examples illustrate this point. Child-hood vaccination confers protection against many potentially lethal infections, yet some parents object to it on the grounds of the real (if rare) risk of side-effects. Fluoridation of the public water supply, a measure that is known to reduce the frequency of dental caries, is regarded by some vociferous oppo-nents as 'mass compulsory medication'. The physical punishment of children, that is likely (in some cases at least) to harm the psychological and physical health of the recipients, is still practised by many parents and carers around the world in the face of near-universal expert disapproval and in breach of the UN Convention on the Rights of the Child as well as the domestic laws of an increasing number of countries. Many people strongly resent this type of intru-sion of governmental policy on the cherished rights of individuals, families and groups. And the clash of values is especially sharpened in times of crisis or large-scale disaster, when public health authorities may be able to invoke the power either of the state or the 'international community' without consulting any of the individuals or communities affected.

Furthermore, public health interventions may not benefit all members of a community equally and this differential impact may be hard to predict. The result is that individuals may be unable to weigh the likely costs against the benefits of an intervention. Many public health measures are aimed at the whole population, only a minority of whom may be at high risk. The measures are effective because they bring about relatively modest changes in large num-bers of people who are at low or medium risk of the disorder in question. The cumulative impact on the population is greater than would be the case were only the small number of people at high risk to be targeted. This 'prevention paradox' (Rose 1981) is a difficult concept to explain to the general public and to politicians. Three examples are reducing the salt content of food to prevent high blood pressure, the fortification of flour with folate to prevent neural tube defects, and the heavy taxation of alcohol and tobacco to reduce consumption of those substances. All of these policies are vigorously opposed, not just by the industries affected but also by large sections of the media and the public who feel that such approaches unfairly penalise people who are unlikely to suffer the disorders in question. They bring into direct confrontation two philosophi-cal value systems – libertarianism and health promotion – that may struggle to find common ground. They epitomise the contrasting, and sometimes irrec-oncilable, perspectives of individualistic and population-based approaches to health improvement.

Ethical dilemmas are unavoidable in public health and there is no consensus on the best methods for resolving them (Wikler and Cash 2009). The choices that have to be made may be momentous and often hinge on the allocation of money, personnel, time or energy – whether, for example, to devote resources to the treatment or prevention of a disease, to children or adults, or to one community rather than another. Poorer communities and groups suffer greater ill health than affluent ones and should, logically, benefit from resource allocation that discriminates in their favour. The evidence, however, suggests that wealthier and better educated sections of the population are more likely to take advantage of health promotion information, services and programmes (Hart 1971). Based on projected estimates of probable health gain, such interventions, if they are to achieve optimal impact, should be delivered primarily to richer rather than poorer people yet the ethics of such a strategy are plainly contentious.

Particular problems arise in relation to the assignment of responsibility when several individuals or agencies undertake public health action collectively. The principle of community empowerment may seem uncontroversial and indeed desirable yet some strongly held communal values may prove incompatible with ethical public health practice, such as when public health practitioners attempt to eradicate female genital mutilation in the face of intense local opposition. Cultural norms that uphold the subjugation of women and the maltreatment of the mentally ill, or justify discrimination against ethnic, sexual or religious minorities, may collide with the public health imperatives of social justice and equitable healthcare. Where conflicts of this type arise, sensitive but firm public health advocacy and diplomacy are required. Explicit reference to international treaties (such as the United Nations Convention on Human Rights), to which most countries have committed themselves, at least in principle, may sometimes help to diffuse tension.

Why public health needs ethical standards

It should not be forgotten that ethics intersect with public health in a bidirectional manner (Beyrer 2007, Mann 1995). Ethically untenable circumstances and practices (such as interpersonal violence, political repression and corruption, social inequality or discrimination based on gender, ethnicity, faith or age) may harbour serious public health implications. These may take many forms such as increasing the risk of death, disability or illness, or causing unnecessary suffering. And public health interventions (such as smoking bans or legislation requiring the wearing of car seatbelts) may sometimes appear to conflict with ethical, legal or political norms as set out by various national or international codes of practice. The position may be summarised as follows: ethics and public health interact with each other in ways that are not always predictable or harmonious.

The slow, inadequate and sometimes counterproductive international response to the global HIV/AIDS pandemic that has killed tens of millions of people has generated heated debate around the ethical failures of the global public health community. Citing the negative experience of that disaster, Cohen *et al* (2007) have argued that an ethical dimension is critical to public health for three reasons. First, all public health interventions should conform to the highest ethical standards since civil societies, by definition, are bounded by implicit moral rules and practices as well as by more formal laws and regulations. Second, healthcare professionals should conduct themselves within a framework of professional ethics akin to the well-established codes of practice that are an accepted feature of clinical medicine. Third, good ethics generally make good policy and practice. The ethical principle of fairness, for example, translates well into the central public health aspiration to reduce health inequalities and to ensure the dignified treatment of all human beings.

A POSSIBLE FRAMEWORK FOR PUBLIC HEALTH ETHICS

If public health is not merely clinical medicine on a large scale, it follows that the ethical aspects of public health are not merely the ethics of clinical medicine applied to populations. A framework specifically designed for public health ethics is required. Kass (2001) has suggested a six-step approach to considering ethics in public health proposals. The six steps may be expressed as a series of questions.

1 What are the public health goals of the proposed intervention?
2 How effective is the proposed intervention likely to be?
3 What is known about the potential burdens or harms arising from the proposed intervention?
4 Does the proposed intervention represent the least burdensome approach?
5 Is the proposed intervention likely to be implemented fairly?
6 How can the public health benefits and accompanying burdens of the proposed intervention be balanced?

The codification of ethical principles into professional standards is an important mechanism for establishing the credibility of and enhancing public trust in that profession's practitioners. There have been various attempts by professional bodies to codify standards for public health practitioners, whether or not they are medically qualified (and therefore subject, in addition, to medical codes of practice). The American Public Health Association (www.apha.org/), for example, has published a public health code of ethics that emphasises:

➤ the prevention of disease
➤ a respect for the rights of individuals
➤ a commitment to working with communities and diverse groups
➤ the need for an evidence-based and multidisciplinary, multisectoral approach
➤ the need to enhance the physical and social environment.

The UK Faculty of Public Health, the standard-setting body for multidisciplinary public health in that country, echoes some of the APHA sentiments in offering ethical guidance to its members. It asserts that public health practice should be equitable, empowering, effective, evidence based, fair and inclusive. These standards are important for training and professional development. Equally, they provide an essential means whereby the public can hold public health practitioners to account.

LEGAL ASPECTS OF PUBLIC HEALTH

Legislation, backed by police enforcement powers, has been a linchpin of public health action for many centuries. Public health authorities are often vested with legally enforceable powers of quarantine, for example, though recourse to such action is generally rare. The legal basis for these powers may be traced back to the early days of public health in Europe when medical officers of health were granted statutory responsibilities to investigate and control outbreaks of infectious diseases. Later, further health protection duties were added, backed by legislation, and included food safety and hygiene, aspects of pollution control, consumer product safety and even slum clearance.

Today, public health practice has extended into other areas of law and its enforcement, notably in the fields of tobacco and alcohol advertising, marketing, sales and licensing. A major new piece of legislation in many countries has banned smoking in indoor public places. Simultaneously, public health practice has become increasingly constrained by legislation designed to protect individuals from harassment, maltreatment, discrimination, disclosure of medical records and other possible violations of human rights. These well-intentioned laws have had both positive and negative effects. On the one hand, they have strengthened personal human rights. Unfortunately, in public health terms, they have sometimes proved counterproductive in that they have discouraged or severely curtailed many previously useful epidemiological activities such as disease surveillance and health services research. They may also, paradoxically, have deprived large numbers of people of the benefits of public health advances through the unnecessarily restrictive interpretation of laws and regulations designed to protect the public from harm.

In addition to domestic law, some international legal treaties have been drafted, several of which (such as the UN Convention on the Rights of the Child) have been mentioned earlier. These have sought to enshrine the right to good health in a manner that obliges governments to reinforce or initiate legislation to protect and promote the health of their populations. Their ultimate effectiveness depends on the willingness of governments to abide by them and to initiate or amend domestic legislation accordingly. In some cases, a more stringent and legally enforceable approach to transnational legislation and regulation has been adopted. The European Union, for example, has introduced a raft of legislation relating to consumer products and services that places a binding commitment on member states to comply fully under the terms of the relevant EU treaties.

REFERENCES

Beyrer C. Human rights and the health of populations. In: Beyrer C, Pizer HF, editors. *Public Health and Human Rights: evidence-based approaches.* Baltimore: Johns Hopkins University Press; 2007.

Cohen J, Kass N, Beyrer C. Human rights and public health ethics: responding to the global HIV/AIDS pandemic. In: Beyrer C, Pizer HF, editors. *Public Health and Human Rights: evidence-based approaches.* Baltimore: Johns Hopkins University Press; 2007.

Gillon R. Medical ethics: four principles plus attention to scope. *BMJ.* 1994; **309**: 184–8.

Hart JT. The inverse care law. *Lancet.* 1971; **1**: 405–12.

Kass N. An ethics framework for public health. *Am J Public Health.* 2001; **91**: 1776–82.

Mann J. Human rights and the new public health. *Health Hum Rights.* 1995; 1(3): 229–33.

Rose G. Strategy of prevention: lessons from cardiovascular disease. *BMJ.* 1981; **282**: 1847–51.

Scott J, Weir DG, Kirke PN. Prevention of neural tube defects with folic acid a success but ... *Q J Med.* 1994; **87**: 705–7.

Wikler D, Cash R. Ethical issues. In: Beaglehole R, Bonita R, editors. *Global Public Health: a new era.* 2nd ed. Oxford: Oxford University Press; 2009.

CHAPTER 15

What does the future hold?

CHANGING EPIDEMIOLOGY OF HEALTH AND DISEASE

As new threats to health emerge and the pattern of diseases evolves, so must the public health response. Bringing about major change in global public health policies and practices is a colossal task akin to setting a new course for the metaphorical oil tanker. The process is a complex one that requires long-term planning and realistic time scales. Horizon scanning is important for detecting and responding to emerging future threats to global health. Crystal balls are notoriously unreliable for predicting the future. A few key demographic and epidemiological trends are, however, likely to continue for the foreseeable future.

The demographic and epidemiological transitions will occur in many poorer countries. The sustainability transition has begun in some parts of the world. All of these will generate opportunities and challenges in ways that can, at least in part, be predicted. The longer life expectancy and ageing of populations will lead to rises in morbidity and burdens on healthcare. There will be a shift in the distribution of deaths from younger to older age groups along with a changing pattern of deaths from communicable diseases and nutritional disorders to chronic diseases (such as cardiovascular diseases and cancer) and trauma. Falling birth rates, below replacement level in many countries, will produce a rising dependency ratio – the ratio of those aged 0–14 and 65+ to those aged 15–65 – with consequences for social services and healthcare. Increasing the statutory retirement age might succeed, in some countries, in holding down the dependency ratio at least for a while.

Healthcare systems are bound to struggle to cope with the impact of population ageing and the associated rising burden of disease. On the other hand, older age is becoming healthier, and it appears that proximity to death rather than age is the determinant of increased healthcare costs, the so-called compression of morbidity (Fries 2003). The increasing complexity of healthcare, especially for previously fatal chronic diseases such as diabetes, cancer and AIDS, will inevitably increase costs. That will pose a formidable challenge in the face of the current global economic downturn. Set against this are other parallel developments. Healthcare costs may fall with the invention of new diagnostic and therapeutic technologies that can be operated by family doctors and community nurses. And rising rates of hospital-acquired infection may act as a negative incentive to hospitalisation and promote the further expansion of community care.

There will be several important changes in the pattern of disease in the coming decades. The Global Burden of Disease study indicates the likely nature of these epidemiological trends. As Figure 15.1 shows, global disability-adjusted life-years (DALYs) are projected to decrease over time by about 10%, from 1.53 billion in 2004 to 1.36 billion in 2030 (Mathers *et al* 2008). The overall projected DALY decline per capita is projected at 30%, largely driven by economic growth in the projection model. This is a remarkable figure given the expected population increase of 25% in that time scale. The causal pattern is also expected to change, with Group 1 (infectious) disorders expected to halve from around 40% in 2004 to 20% of DALYs in 2030. Respiratory disorders, diarrhoeal diseases and HIV/AIDS are expected to decline steeply. The corollary is that the Group 2 (non-communicable) causes are expected to increase to 66% of DALYs and to dominate the burden in all regions. In 2030, the three leading causes of DALYs are projected to be unipolar depressive disorders, ischaemic heart disease and road traffic accidents. Indeed, injuries as a whole seem likely to climb the international burden of disease league table. Injury-related mortality is expected to rise up the burden of disease league table in

2004 Disease or Injury	As % of total DALYs	Rank	Rank	As % of total DALYs	2030 Disease or Injury
Lower respiratory infections	6.2	1	1	6.2	Unipolar depressive disorders
Diarrhoeal diseases	4.8	2	2	5.5	Ischaemic heart disease
Unipolar depressive disorders	4.3	3	3	4.9	Road traffic accidents
Ischaemic heart disease	4.1	4	4	4.3	Cerebrovascular disease
HIV/AIDS	3.8	5	5	3.8	COPD
Cerebrovascular disease	3.1	6	6	3.2	Lower respiratory infections
Prematurity and low birth weight	2.9	7	7	2.9	Hearing loss, adult onset
Birth asphyxia and birth trauma	2.7	8	8	2.7	Refractive errors
Road traffic accidents	2.7	9	9	2.5	HIV/AIDS
Neonatal infections and other	2.7	10	10	2.3	Diabetes mellitus
COPD	2.0	13	11	1.9	Neonatal infections and other
Refractive errors	1.8	14	12	1.9	Prematurity and low birth weight
Hearing loss, adult onset	1.8	15	15	1.9	Birth asphyxia and birth trauma
Diabetes mellitus	1.3	19	18	1.6	Diarrhoeal diseases

Figure 15.1 Global Burden of Disease study projections 2004–30.
Source: Mathers *et al* (2008).

the coming decades, from around 5 million deaths to over 8 million by 2030, when the number of DALYs attributable to injuries will far exceed those from cardiovascular or respiratory disease. Younger age groups will suffer in particular. Adolescents and young men, especially those living in low-income countries, have a higher risk from road casualties, interpersonal violence, suicide and war.

EPIDEMIOLOGICAL TRENDS WILL BE INFLUENCED BY THE ECONOMY AND ENVIRONMENT

Three specific areas to which public health practitioners and policy makers will have to devote increasing attention are globalisation, climate change and group violence.

Globalisation

Globalisation describes the process whereby people and countries become increasingly interconnected and interdependent. It comprises two inter-related components: the opening of international borders to an increasingly rapid flow of goods, services, finance, people and ideas; and the changing national international and institutional policies that promote these flows (Sharma and Atri 2010). Major drivers of globalisation include technological advances, the reduced costs of making transactions, and the increased mobility of capital. Its impact has already been enormous and has been felt across many dimensions, notably economic (trade liberalisation and deregulation), technological (telecommunications and transport) and political (redistribution of power from states to interstate bodies).

Globalisation is a term that polarises opinion. On one side are the enthusiasts who regard it as an opportunity for improving global trade, increasing information exchange, accelerating skills development and promoting health. On the other are the sceptics who argue that the advocates of globalisation usually have a vested interest because it perpetuates the fundamentally exploitative relationship between rich and poor countries. An intermediate position views globalisation as an inevitable consequence of economic and technological progress which should be recognised as harbouring the potential for both good and ill. Almost everyone agrees, however, that the phenomenon is real, irreversible and extremely significant for global health. The effects of globalisation on global health are undoubtedly both positive and negative, a confusing reality that tends to blunt the confrontational nature of the debate.

The increased movement of goods and people magnifies the risks arising from infections (such as H5N1 avian influenza) and other health risks to which people are exposed. This can occur either directly, through the marketing of potentially hazardous consumer products, or indirectly, via the expansion of transport and other infrastructures that pose a potential threat to human health. Among the most serious public health threats that may be attributed to globalisation are:

➤ emerging diseases
➤ nuclear, chemical and biological terrorism
➤ environmental disruption
➤ economic instability
➤ international crises and humanitarian emergencies.

A related development is urbanisation and that too is a double-edged sword. Specialised healthcare (such as trauma care) is more easily organised and delivered in urban than in rural settings, and increases the uptake and impact of preventive measures (such as immunisation) and reduces case fatality rates (through access to more effective therapies). Offsetting these benefits to some extent is the proliferation of urban slums in response to mass migration towards cities, creating new, unfamiliar and sometimes lethal health hazards – most obviously associated with road traffic – to families and children.

Some of the effects of globalisation affect population health indirectly. Two striking examples are the recent economic crisis and the information revolution. The increasing interconnectedness of the world economy means that an economic slump in one region has immediate repercussions elsewhere, as vividly illustrated by the international banking failure of 2008. Though magnified by a recessionary tendency that was already under way, the collapse of Lehman Brothers, a major US bank, triggered a sequence of events that engulfed all the world's markets, reduced financial liquidity, depressed national economies and prompted massive public expenditure. The last of these led to equally huge cuts in services and rising inflation. The effects of these trends on health remain uncertain but most are likely to be negative. Early indications are that economic growth may have stalled in those low-income countries that were showing promising signs of closing the gap on their more affluent counterparts. Previous economic crises in Asia and elsewhere appear to have contributed to rising rates of low birthweight, child mortality, malnutrition and stunting, as well as higher unemployment, reduced family income and a deterioration in a range of other health and quality-of-life indicators (Patel 2009). As unemployment rates rise, suicide rates tend to follow (Stuckler *et al* 2011). The economic downturn may also cause political instability, military coups, conflict and human rights abuses.

All these adverse consequences of recession and poor economic growth are expected to become increasingly manifest in the coming years though the time scale is uncertain. This means that the past trend of steadily widening social inequalities in health, both between and within countries, is unlikely to be reversed and will continue to preoccupy public health professionals and governments for the foreseeable future. They will also undermine progress in improving global health.

The globalisation of information through the 24-hour news media, the internet and numerous social networking sites such as Facebook and Twitter has resulted in a rapid increase in international communication. The more rapid dissemination of information around the world is generally beneficial in raising awareness of health and how to promote and protect it from avoidable threats. It has also greatly heightened awareness throughout the world about egregious military behaviour, human rights abuses and other significant events. This is generally beneficial in the sense that public opinion, either generally or operating through lobby groups, can be mobilised more easily to exert pressure on corrupt governments and repressive politicians to change their behaviour. The 'Arab Spring' of 2011 is a notable manifestation of internet-generated political upheavals of this type. On the other hand, this carries risks. Individuals or groups with malign political goals are more easily able to exploit the output of the mass media to disseminate highly selective or biased information, extremist propaganda and even incitement to violence with much greater speed and effectiveness than in the past.

Climate change

The environmental phenomenon that is probably generating most current concern about its global public health impact (both direct and indirect) is climate change. Various atmospheric factors, notably increased CO_2 emissions, appear to be contributing to a protracted process of climate change, though the occurrence of abrupt and highly dangerous disturbances is also possible. The scientific debate is not yet fully settled but the general consensus is that climate change is real, manmade and amenable to intervention. According to the Intergovernmental Panel on Climate Change (2007), temperatures are steadily rising in all continents. The global average annual temperature is predicted to rise by between 1.1°C and 6.4°C from the late 20th to the late 21st century. Although this will convey some health benefits (such as a decline in hypothermia deaths), these will be greatly outweighed by the more significant negative ones (*see* Chapter 2). The latter will be extremely dangerous to human health if the temperature rises by 2°C and potentially catastrophic if the rise is higher than this level.

Among the expected adverse effects of climate change that have direct consequences for human health (Griffiths *et al* 2009) are extreme weather events (especially heatwaves, droughts, floods and storms, all of which can result in deaths, physical injuries and mental ill health), poor air quality and a high pollen count, reduced food safety due to warmer temperatures, and increased exposure to ultraviolet radiation. An increase in vector-borne infections, such as malaria, Lyme disease and dengue fever, will also ensue. Indirect effects include rising food prices, mass migration, long-term unemployment, increasing poverty, political instability and international conflict. As is so often the case, the adverse health effects of climate change will disproportionately affect poorer countries and particularly people living in coastal, mountainous or polar regions.

Even when the meteorological evidence becomes more reliable, as is likely to happen in the coming years, the precise impact of climate change on human health will be difficult to predict. The causal pathways are complex and intersect with many other environmental risks, including stratospheric ozone depletion, disruption of food supplies, depleted sources of freshwater and the loss of biodiversity. The first priority will be for public health investigators, climatatologists, geographers, statisticians and other scientists to work together to evaluate the risks and develop strategies to implement countermeasures. Some of these will be short term (such as preparing heatwave plans) while others will be long term (such as reducing CO_2 emissions). As the stakes are so high, the 'prudence principle' demands that we take action sooner rather than later. Some of the most effective interventions are already available and are being applied, albeit inadequately, through national policies and international treaties.

The UN Framework on Climate Change (of 1992), the World Meteorological Organization and the UN Environment Programme (that created the Intergovernmental Panel on Climate Change), and the Kyoto Protocol of 1997 have all addressed the challenge of climate change, with mixed results. The World Bank (2010) noted that from 1997 to 2005, energy emissions grew by 24% and criticised the Kyoto Protocol for providing minimal assistance to developing countries to assist in implementation. The USA refused to sign the treaty, citing unhappiness with the virtual exemption of major polluters such as India and China from stringent caps on carbon emissions. Many signatory states have paid lip service only to the Protocol while indulging in diversionary anti-American rhetoric. From a public health perspective, these disappointments should not delay action. What is needed is a systematic framework of primary, secondary and tertiary preventive measures within which to plan, implement and monitor national and global interventions (Griffiths *et al* 2009).

Group (collective) violence

Scale of the problem of group violence

Every year, hundreds of thousands (and sometimes many more) people die as a result of group violence. Reliable data are elusive, first, because many countries (especially in the developing world) lack sophisticated routine data systems, and, second, because of bias. Bias and selective reporting are notorious problems when violence is committed in a political context by organised groups or states because of their desire to vindicate themselves and to manipulate public opinion. The World Health Organization (WHO) tends to place great store on data reported by humanitarian organisations such as Amnesty International and Human Rights Watch, ignoring the inconvenient fact that these non-governmental organisations (NGOs) may also be subject to external and internal pressures that may severely bias the information they publish.

Group violence has blighted human existence since records began. It is impossible to calculate the vast number of lives lost from this cause throughout history. Group violence is a particular cause for concern in poorer countries due to their greater likelihood of experiencing war, civil unrest and internecine conflict. Terrorism is a growing preoccupation of many countries, rich and poor. Since the September 11th 2001 attacks on the USA, it has become clear that well-funded terrorist groups, many of which proclaim political or religious objectives that cannot under any circumstances be realised, have the motivation and occasionally the means to inflict mass casualties on civilian populations.

If a public health approach to unintentional injuries is a fairly new phenomenon, its application to violence of all kinds, and group violence in particular, is extremely rare. An overtly public health perspective on group (or collective or mass) violence and its prevention has recently begun to be articulated. Dahlberg and Krug (2002) have defined collective violence as:

> the instrumental use of violence by people who identify themselves as members of a group – whether this group is transitory or has a more permanent identity – against another group or set of individuals, in order to achieve political, economic or social objectives. (Reproduced by permission of WHO)

The WHO describes three levels of group violence:
➤ wars, terrorism or other violent interstate political conflicts
➤ state-perpetrated violence such as genocide and torture
➤ organised violent crime such as banditry and gang warfare.

This may be paraphrased as political violence, state-sponsored repressive violence and mass criminal violence. Of these, only warfare has, in some circumstances, a legal basis and this relates both to its declaration and conduct. Legal justification for the declaration of war resides in the United Nations Charter (with Articles 42 and 51 of Chapter Seven setting out the criteria). Once war has been declared, its conduct should comply with the Geneva Convention of 1949. The interpretation of these documents is often highly contentious.

Perhaps the most extreme, horrifying and inexplicable type of mass violence is genocide. This is defined by the 1948 Convention on the Prevention and Punishment of the Crime of Genocide (published in the wake of the Nazi Holocaust) as: 'Any ... acts committed with intent to destroy, in whole or in part, a national, ethnical, racial or religious group'. The Convention was regarded by its authors as a tool designed to ensure that a repeat of the Nazi

Holocaust would never again be tolerated by the international community. In the succeeding decades, events in Cambodia, Rwanda, Darfur and elsewhere demonstrated the naivety of this belief.

How can collective violence be prevented?

Despite its catastrophic effects on the health and wellbeing of entire communities, ethnic groups and countries, group or collective violence (including genocide) appears to have received surprisingly little attention from the global public health community. Krug *et al* (2002) documented the wide range of adverse consequences of collective violence, including war, terrorism and torture, on population health. They proposed several strategies for preventing collective violence, including reducing its potential by modifying risk factors, promoting the compliance of countries with international agreements, responding quickly and effectively to outbreaks of collective violence through political and humanitarian action, deploying UN peace-keeping measures in conflict zones, harnessing the influence of the healthcare sector to document and respond to violence, and carefully recording and disseminating information, including that generated by research, on violent conflicts around the world.

A sophisticated public health approach to reduce the incidence of collective violence needs to take account of the modifiability of risk factors, the international organisational and legal context, the state of public opinion, the role of the health sector, the importance of careful documentation, and research. The paucity of research means that the evidence base for intervention is extremely limited. Furthermore, history has shown that cynical political calculations by individual countries, groups of countries or leaders tend to trump proposals for countermeasures that are motivated by humanitarian concerns.

RESPONDING TO FUTURE CHALLENGES

Beaglehole and Bonita (2009) have called for a reinvigorated public health response to the key challenges facing the discipline: the daunting global health context, the weakness of the public health workforce and infrastructure, and the need to clarify and broaden the scope of public health practice. They envisage public health practitioners playing a leading role in:

➤ responding to immediate health crises such as pandemics of diseases and environmental disruption
➤ reforming the health sector in a manner that improves population health and enhances equity
➤ promoting intersectoral actions for health improvement.

To fulfil these roles, these authors suggest that public health research, training and practice will have to be adequately resourced, policy makers will need to draw on the findings of public health research to ensure that the most effective policies are supported, and public health practitioners will have to provide timely and relevant information from surveillance systems that take account of regional and global perspectives. Finally, they call for the values of public health to be made explicit, and for mutually reinforcing interactions to be established between public health practitioners, clinicians and the communities they serve.

Both vertical and horizontal public health interventions will be needed

Given the uncertainties surrounding future predictions, particularly because of the likely continuing inadequacy of knowledge generation through interventional research, any medium- or long-term planning designed to address public health challenges that have yet to materialise must be tentative. That does not mean we should do nothing. On the contrary, the more we try to anticipate trends, the greater the prospects of success in confronting them. Our strategic response to future uncertainty should be twofold. First, we should recognise that many current programmes are well placed to respond to the changing public health landscape. We should continue to advocate and sustain existing *vertical interventions* aimed at specific disorders or goals. These have proven effective in the past and they will certainly continue to play a crucial role in the future. The 'big three' infectious diseases – AIDS, malaria and tuberculosis – will be with us for the foreseeable future, as will most of the other causes of contemporary mortality and morbidity, and will demand persistent public health attention. Second, we should invest greater efforts in developing and evaluating *horizontal interventions* and approaches, including an overarching global strategy of the kind proposed in the Appendix. Adopting horizontal perspectives will optimise our chances of solving a variety of emerging problems, many of which may be traced to a single common pathway.

Under the 'environmental' rubric, global warming and related phenomena will be a high priority. Addressing the threat of climate change will require humanity to undergo the 'sustainability transition' (*see* Chapter 2) towards a low-carbon, resource-conserving macro-economy (McMichael *et al* 2006). The public health community, including healthcare practitioners, will be expected to play a leading role in this enterprise (Griffiths *et al* 2009). Promoting sustainability will demand a combination of strategies, including seeking to reduce greenhouse gas emissions (mitigation through primary prevention) and reducing the impact of climate change on populations (adaptation through secondary and tertiary prevention). A key part of this process will be the fostering of community resilience to optimise the prospects for successful adaptation. We can enhance resilience by modelling likely future scenarios based on varying assumptions (e.g. a 3°C versus a 1°C temperature rise), by establishing effective environmental and health monitoring systems, by co-ordinating environmental, energy and health policies, by strengthening general public health capacity (including disaster preparedness), and by conducting evaluational research to determine the most appropriate and effective environmental responses.

Healthcare has a place in the public health response

McKeown (1976) argued that healthcare made a very limited impact on improving mortality rates in the 20th century. More recent evidence suggests that medical interventions can add several years to life expectancy (Bunker *et al* 1995, Hypertension Detection and Follow-up Program Co-operative Group 1987). McKee (2006) argues forcefully that healthcare makes a real contribution to public health and that 'about half of the improvement in life expectancy in western European countries over the past three decades can be attributed to the impact of healthcare'. The other half is attributable, in large part, to risk factor (notably smoking) reduction, some of which, at least, was achieved through the (mainly primary) healthcare system.

It seems, then, that clinical interventions may have the potential to reduce mortality from coronary heart disease (and perhaps other diseases) by more than half (Critchley and Capewell 2003). Even pandemics of infectious diseases, such as AIDS, may be confronted effectively through the merging of preventive and therapeutic approaches (*Economist* 2011). The scope for further improvements in public health arising from scientific advances combined with evidence-based healthcare practice remains considerable. Genomics has failed to deliver the promised major public health benefits to date but may yet do so in the future.

McKee (2006) argues for a new model of healthcare investment that goes beyond the traditional production function. He proposes that output be maximised by an optimal combination of people (human capital), human relationships (social capital), facilities and equipment (physical capital) and knowledge (intellectual capital). All of these require a long-term approach (sustainability) and organisational competence (management). He elaborates these ideas as (and I paraphrase):

➤ developing an appropriate mix of skills in the healthcare workforce that takes account of rapidly changing roles, and enhancing all professionals' ability to absorb the increasing volume of new knowledge (human capital)

➤ reconfiguring facilities such as hospitals that will enable them to adapt quickly to new challenges, and adopting a more strategic approach to health technology and its applications (physical capital)

➤ developing new knowledge systems in which the generation of information (by researchers), its synthesis (by knowledge brokers or translational researchers) and implementation (by research-aware practitioners) are integrated into healthcare systems (intellectual capital)

➤ enhancing the healthcare environment in a way that nurtures positive staff relationships, trust and communication to optimise outcomes and lower costs (social capital)

➤ sustaining all of these investments over time and ensuring flexibility in the light of emerging problems and changing evidence about effectiveness and efficiency (sustainability)

➤ applying high-quality financial and organisational management, including the creation of zones of stability in an era of change, throughout the healthcare sector (management).

In 2010, the UN launched its Global Strategy for Women's and Children's Health (United Nations 2010) in an attempt to revitalise progress towards meeting the Millennium Development Goals. Around $40 billion has been committed until 2015. Much of this will be spent on training health workers, at least 3.5 million of whom will be needed to fill the current gap in capacity, according to the Global Health Workforce Alliance, especially in low-income countries. The Alliance calls for the recruitment and training of midwives, birth attendants and community health workers to meet the needs of maternal and child health.

FUTURE GLOBAL PUBLIC HEALTH PRIORITIES

The future orientation of public health will have to change if it is to remain relevant. Its scope, activities, training and research will be obliged to address several concerns that have been relatively neglected by the public health community and are bound to grow in importance. Several of these have been discussed earlier in this book. Global public health capacity urgently needs replenishing and nurturing, and that means expanding training programmes and providing better career structures for new recruits to the field. Practitioners will need a more supportive infrastructure within which to work and that will require greater resource allocation and administrative support for public health agencies and departments. Given the key role of information in public health planning, strengthening national and transnational vital statistical agencies and health surveillance systems is clearly a high priority. Encouraging more research into the most effective and efficient approaches to health improvement, in the broadest sense, is essential for generating the knowledge that is needed to inform the global public health effort. Despite their ubiquitous scarcity, we must ensure that sufficient resources are allocated, albeit with careful mechanisms for governance and accountability, to meet the pressing health, educational and social needs of the entire global population, especially those trapped in severe poverty. Finally, inspirational and competent leadership will always be necessary to cope with future turbulence.

Can we prioritise this daunting agenda? Here is a reminder of my 'shortlist' of six global public health priorities for immediate action, selected from the proposed 'horizontal' global public health strategy (*see* the Appendix), outlined in Chapter 10.

1 Work with others to eliminate poverty and inequity.
2 Focus on creating a healthy, safe and sustainable environment.
3 Start early in the lifecourse to prevent disease and improve health.
4 Adopt a horizontal strategic framework for global public health.
5 Improve global health data.
6 Boost public health capacity.

All of these will demand relentless attention in the coming decades. But the global public health agenda is enormous and will have to be kept under continuous review. While it is impossible to cover all eventualities, some emerging concerns are becoming visible on the horizon. To try to anticipate just a few of those, I propose, in addition to the above list, six further urgent priorities for attention and action, all of which have been highlighted intermittently throughout this book.

1 Investigate and promote wellbeing, mental health and quality of life.
2 Nurture salutogenesis, including boosting social capital, resilience and resistance.
3 Seek professional mechanisms to balance human rights and responsibilities.
4 Confront violence, terrorism and conflict as public health challenges.
5 Exploit more fully the public health role of healthcare systems and practitioners.
6 Resolve the tension, through strong leadership, between competing priorities.

That list of six top strategic actions and six further topics for urgent attention represents an ambitious agenda in itself (Box 15.1). Others will doubtless be able to offer their own suggestions in response to the emergence of new diseases, disorders and risk factors. There is clearly no 'right' or 'wrong' list and it is up to individual practitioners, national governments and international organisations to formulate their own proposals for action. All constructive ideas are worthy of consideration, discussion and ranking as a set of proposed priorities. What is important is that the exercise should be undertaken and an international consensus achieved as quickly as possible.

TWO QUESTIONS

At this point, I would urge all readers who have patiently stayed the course to ask themselves two questions. First, on the basis of the evidence and arguments

BOX 15.1 *Proposed list of 12 areas for horizontal global public health action*

Top priorities for immediate attention
➤ Work with others to eliminate poverty and inequity.
➤ Focus on creating a healthy, safe and sustainable environment.
➤ Start early in the lifecourse to prevent disease and improve health.
➤ Adopt a horizontal strategic framework for global public health.
➤ Improve global health data.
➤ Boost public health capacity.

Other urgent priorities
➤ Investigate and promote wellbeing, mental health and quality of life.
➤ Nurture salutogenesis, including boosting social capital, resilience and resistance.
➤ Seek professional mechanisms to balance human rights and responsibilities.
➤ Confront violence, terrorism and conflict as public health challenges.
➤ Exploit more fully the public health role of healthcare systems and practitioners.
➤ Resolve the tension, through strong leadership, between competing priorities.

presented in this book, am I persuaded that we are facing (or are about to face) a crisis in global public health? Second, do I agree with the strategic priorities for action proposed, either within the shortlist of 12 topics or in the form of the comprehensive horizontal strategic framework presented in the Appendix?

I believe that the act of pondering these questions is likely to be more productive than arguing over the answers. Readers will vary widely in their responses. Achieving a consensus view is an unrealistic objective. What is more important is that we (that is, all who are concerned with global public health) should agree that the case for action is overwhelming. The global public health community has a responsibility to weigh the evidence, discuss the possible content of the strategies and haggle over resources and time scales. But as human beings, we have an even greater responsibility: to participate in the debate, to pressurise (where we can) our governments to act to improve and protect population health, and to hold them to account when they decline.

REFERENCES

Beaglehole R, Bonita R, editors. *Global Public Health: a new era*. Oxford: Oxford University Press; 2009. pp.185–207.

Bunker JP, Frazier HS, Mosteller F. The role of medical care in determining health: creating an inventory of benefits. In: Amick BC, Levine AR, Tarlov AR, *et al*, editors. *Society and Health*. New York: Oxford University Press; 1995.

Critchley JA, Capewell S. Substantial potential for reductions in coronary heart disease mortality in the UK through changes in risk factor levels. *J Epidemiol Commun Health*. 2003; **57**: 243–7.

Dahlberg LL, Krug EG. Violence – a global public health problem. In: Krug EG, Dahlberg LL, Mercy JA, *et al*, editors. *World Report on Violence and Health*. Geneva: World Health Organization; 2002. pp. 1–56.

Economist. The end of AIDS? (leader). *The Economist*. 2011; June 4th; 13.

Fries JF. Measuring and monitoring success in compressing morbidity. *Ann Intern Med*. 2003; **139**: 455–9.

Griffiths J, Rao M, Adshead F, *et al*. *The Health Practitioner's Guide to Climate Change: diagnosis and cure*. London: Earthscan; 2009.

Hypertension Detection and Follow-up Program Co-operative Group. Education level and 5 year all-cause mortality in the HDFP. *Hypertension*. 1987; **9**: 641–6.

Intergovernmental Panel on Climate Change. *Climate Change 2007 – the science of climate change*. Cambridge: Cambridge University Press; 2007.

Krug EG, Dahlberg LL, Mercy JA, *et al*, editors. *World Report on Violence and Health*. Geneva: World Health Organization; 2002.

Mathers C, Boerma T, Fat Ma D. *The Global Burden of Disease. 2004 update*. Geneva: World Health Organization; 2008.

McKee M. The future. In: Marinker M, editor. *Constructive Conversations about Health*. Oxford: Radcliffe Publishing; 2006.

McKeown T. *The Role of Medicine: dream, mirage or nemesis?* London: Nuffield Provincial Hospitals Trust; 1976.

McMichael AJ, Woodruff RE, Hales S. Climate change and human health: present and future risks. *Lancet*. 2006; **367**: 859–69.

Patel M. Economic crisis and children: an overview for East Asia and the Pacific. *Global Soc Policy*. 2009; **9**: 33.

Sharma M, Atri A. *Essentials of International Health*. Sudbury, MA: Jones and Bartlett Publishers; 2010.

Stuckler D, Basu S, Suhrcke M, *et al*. Effects of the 2008 recession on health: a first look at European data (letter). *Lancet*. 2011; **378**: 124–5.

United Nations. *Every Woman, Every Child: global strategy for women's and children's health*. 2010. www.un.org/sg/hf/global_strategy_commitments.pdf

World Bank. *World Development Report 2010: development and climate change*. Washington DC: World Bank; 2010.

Section 3 summary

Compliance with public health strategies cannot be taken for granted but can be facilitated by capacity building, promoting networking and collaboration, allocating resources in the form of personnel and finance, incorporating robust performance management systems, and creating an effective administrative infrastructure.

The key attributes of a successful public health delivery system include:

➤ availability of reliable and relevant data on population health
➤ professional and political leadership in public health
➤ coherent planning linked to well-managed, evidence-based frontline programmes
➤ allocation of adequate financial and human resources
➤ deployment of practitioners with appropriate skills
➤ development of capacity through education and training
➤ co-ordination of healthcare and preventive services
➤ careful monitoring of performance and outcomes.

Evaluation is crucial to ensuring effective implementation. Professionals might set about an evaluation in five steps: clarify programme goals, design an evaluation plan, develop and implement a data collection plan, analyse and interpret the data, and use the findings.

The need for translational research is as paramount within public health as it is within clinical disciplines though this is not always acknowledged explicitly. And harnessing the potential of science and technology to the demands of global public health has the potential to secure further breakthroughs in the future. As well as the six top priorities for action outlined earlier, six further priorities for medium- and long-term attention are proposed, giving us an agenda for action.

The *top priorities for immediate action* are:

➤ work with others to eliminate poverty and inequity
➤ focus on creating a healthy, safe and sustainable environment
➤ start early in the lifecourse to prevent disease and improve health
➤ adopt a horizontal strategic framework for global public health
➤ improve global health data
➤ boost public health capacity.

Other *urgent priorities* are:

➤ investigate and promote wellbeing, mental health and quality of life
➤ nurture salutogenesis, including boosting social capital, resilience and resistance
➤ seek professional mechanisms to balance human rights and responsibilities
➤ confront violence, terrorism and conflict as public health challenges
➤ exploit more fully the public health role of healthcare systems and practitioners
➤ resolve the tension, through strong leadership, between competing priorities.

Postscript: key messages of the book

DIAGNOSIS

The underlying premise (or hypothesis) of this book is that the world is facing a serious, prolonged and potentially disastrous public health crisis that is all the more dangerous for its near invisibility. In trying to analyse the nature of the crisis, I have adopted a three-step model – diagnosis, treatment, follow-up – that is broadly analogous to the systematic approach familiar to clinicians. The diagnostic step is especially critical as everything thereafter flows from it.

Making a global health diagnosis is far from straightforward. We have at our disposal a plethora of data but these are incomplete and of dubious quality. Most of the available data describe mortality – the tip of the epidemiological pyramid – while morbidity and disability data are notable for their scarcity. The Global Burden of Disease study has provided us with an unprecedented epidemiological tool for assessing the health of the world's population in a way that permits comparisons between countries and regions across a number of health dimensions.

As with all epidemiological analyses, we can examine population health status in terms of place, time and personal characteristics (or risk factors). There is huge geographical variation in health both between and within countries. To make sense of the changing nature of global health over time, and to respond to it effectively, we have to take account of three phenomena: the demographic, epidemiological and sustainability transitions. And understanding the role and origin of risk factors, such as smoking and drinking, is an essential component of the global health diagnosis.

Health and wealth are intimately related. It is no coincidence that the poorest countries suffer the worst health in the world. On the other hand, poverty exists in all regions and countries of the world. Even the most affluent countries contain pockets of extreme poverty and suffer the adverse health effects of social inequalities. With rising awareness of the damaging effects of these inequalities, researchers, practitioners and policy makers are becoming increasingly preoccupied with ways to overcome them.

While poverty is a key determinant of health, it is far from the only one. Countries that have experienced political turmoil, such as those in the former Soviet Union, have also suffered upturns in premature mortality in ways that seem unrelated to absolute poverty. Moreover, poverty interacts with other risks to health in complex ways that are not yet fully understood. The origins of many disorders of childhood and adult life can be traced to early life, especially to the intrauterine and preschool phases of the life cycle, and several research or aetiological paradigms have been invoked by way of explanation. These include biological, psychosocial and socioeconomic theories that are not necessarily mutually exclusive. Whichever paradigm is favoured at any given moment, the bottom-line message is the same: if we are to understand and improve human health at any age, we have to view health across the entire life cycle, from conception to death, and, additionally, to adopt an intergenerational perspective.

How can we summarise the current state of global health? This is an almost impossible task. We can arrive at an approximate global health diagnosis by juxtaposing two complementary statements. First, we have achieved enormous progress in global health in the last half-century, notably lower child mortality and improved life expectancy in many countries, but the picture is highly variable, with some large regions of the world showing worrying signs of deteriorating health. Second, most of the progress observed up till now may turn out to have been fragile as a result of newly arising threats from shifting demographic patterns, epidemiological setbacks in the control of both communicable and chronic diseases, global environmental disruption, economic stress, political instability and violence.

TREATMENT

Having formulated, as best we can, a global health diagnosis, what can we do to improve matters? Or, more precisely, what should we do over and above the many interventions that are already taking place around the world? Can we devise an intervention or series of countermeasures analogous to the treatment plan prescribed by a clinician to a patient?

Although the scale of the challenge is daunting, that should not deter us from action. On the contrary, it should fire our collective ambition. First and foremost, a global challenge requires a global response. That should be articulated as a global public health strategy. Some of its elements already exist in the texts of international agreements such as the Ottawa Charter (1986) and the Millennium Declaration (2000). While these and similar international endeavours are important, they need to be integrated into a single overarching strategic framework that is currently lacking.

Here is a possible global public health mission statement for our time.

To embrace, at a global level, a form of public health that is holistic in scope and aspires to influence the health of populations with a view to:
- improving and protecting health and wellbeing
- preventing ill health (and the risk of ill health), disability and suffering
- reducing health inequalities between genders, races, social groups, communities and countries
- nurturing an ecologically sustainable environment for future generations.

A strategy contains elements that may either be cross-cutting ('horizontal') or highly focused ('vertical'). Here are five *key principles* that might inform a 'horizontal' global public health strategy.

1 Embrace a holistic view of health and disease on which to base public health responses.
2 Apply a pragmatic evidence-based approach to public health policy making and practice.
3 Adopt a lifecourse perspective on public health analysis and intervention.
4 Create efficient and transparent governance processes for public health action.
5 Strive for a comprehensive strategic overview of public health policy making and practice.

I have formulated a draft horizontal strategy (*see* the Appendix) from which I have selected *six top priorities for immediate horizontal strategic action*. Three are recommendations for specific policy action while three relate to the global public health infrastructure.

The three *policy action* points are:
1 work with others to eliminate absolute poverty and ameliorate relative poverty
2 focus on creating a healthy, safe and sustainable environment
3 start early in the lifecourse to prevent disease and improve health.

The three recommendations for action to improve the *infrastructure* are:
1 adopt a horizontal strategic framework for global public health while continuing to deliver vertical interventions
2 improve routine health data completeness and quality
3 boost public health capacity in the form of personnel, skills and resources.

FOLLOW-UP

Developing strategies is important but will achieve nothing unless the strategies are implemented. (In clinical practice, even patients who appear to agree with the recommendations of healthcare practitioners may fail to implement them.) That is why it is so important, through careful follow-up, to ensure that the prescribed treatment has actually happened. Compliance with public health strategies can be facilitated by capacity building, networking, collaborating, allocating resources in the form of personnel and finance, incorporating robust performance management systems, and creating effective administrative infrastructures. The prospects of success will be greatly enhanced if thought has been given to delivery vehicles, either through the exploitation of existing organisational structures and programmes or by creating new ones.

A list of the key attributes of a successful public health delivery system might include:

➤ availability of reliable and relevant data on population health
➤ professional and political leadership in public health
➤ coherent planning linked to well-managed, evidence-based frontline programmes
➤ allocation of adequate financial and human resources
➤ deployment of practitioners with appropriate skills
➤ development of capacity through education and training
➤ co-ordination of healthcare and preventive services
➤ careful monitoring of performance and outcomes.

Evaluation is crucial to monitoring progress and ensuring effective implementation. Public health professionals might set about evaluation in five steps: clarify programme goals, design an evaluation plan, develop and implement a data collection plan, analyse and interpret the data, and use the findings.

The need for translational research is as paramount within public health as in clinical medicine. Harnessing the potential of science and technology to meet the demands of global public health has the potential to secure further breakthroughs in the future.

The six top priorities for immediate strategic action (listed above under Treatment) are only a starting point for ongoing strategic thinking. Looking to the future, and in an attempt to anticipate emerging public health threats, I have identified six further, longer-term though nevertheless *urgent priorities for strategic action*. These are:

1 investigate and promote wellbeing, mental health and quality of life
2 nurture salutogenesis, including boosting social capital, resilience and resistance
3 seek professional mechanisms to balance human rights and responsibilities
4 confront violence, terrorism and conflict as public health challenges
5 exploit more fully the public health role of healthcare systems and practitioners
6 resolve the tension between competing public health objectives.

THE BOTTOM LINE

The health of the world's population is in a state of constant flux. The overall pattern contains both good and bad news, and the justified satisfaction with improved life expectancy in most countries should be tempered by concern regarding emerging disorders, risk factors and threats. Many professionals, policy makers, agencies and organisations are involved in the multilevel tasks of attempting to clarify the global burden of disease (diagnosis), deciding on the most effective and efficient interventions (treatment) and evaluating the impact of our efforts (follow-up). Together, these represent the three-step public health approach applied to the analysis of global population health and wellbeing.

Because of the massive scale of the challenge, as well as its sheer complexity, everything we say about the state of global health has to be provisional. Both the state of global population health and our array of available, evidence-based countermeasures are constantly changing. We can, however, reasonably characterise our current dilemma as a prolonged crisis. We are far from impotent in our efforts to confront it, however. So what should we do? What is the 'bottom-line' message of this book?

The answer lies in the reinvigoration of the three-step public health approach that is already under way. In particular, we need to redouble our efforts to analyse population health in a manner that promotes evidence-based strategic thinking, both vertical and horizontal. Many excellent vertical programmes are up and running and these should be supported and strengthened. Horizontal strategy development has lagged behind and requires substantial reinforcement. A proposed horizontal strategy for global public health is shown in the Appendix. It represents one possible approach – it is neither the first word on the subject nor will it be the last. If it contributes to an international debate about how we can move forward, strategically, it will have achieved its purpose.

REITERATION: 12 PRIORITIES FOR GLOBAL PUBLIC HEALTH

Distilling all the ideas presented into a set of specific recommendations is not easy and to assume that they will command universal support is unrealistic. Nevertheless, as a contribution to the debate about global public health, here is my shortlist of *12 priorities for action*. The first six, I suggest, demand immediate action, but all demand sustained attention and long-term strategic review.

Six *top priorities for immediate action* are:
1   work with others to eliminate absolute poverty and ameliorate relative poverty
2   focus on creating a healthy, safe and sustainable environment
3   start early in the lifecourse to prevent disease and improve health
4   adopt a horizontal strategic framework for global public health while continuing to deliver vertical interventions

5   improve routine health data completeness and quality
6   boost public health capacity in the form of personnel, skills and resources.

The first three of these top priorities relate to policy actions, the remainder to the global public health infrastructure.

Six further *urgent priorities for action* are:
1   investigate and promote wellbeing, mental health and quality of life
2   nurture salutogenesis, including boosting social capital, resilience and resistance
3   seek professional mechanisms to balance human rights and responsibilities
4   confront violence, terrorism and conflict as public health challenges
5   exploit more fully the public health role of healthcare systems and practitioners
6   resolve the tension between competing public health objectives.

All of these should be viewed in the context of the need to constantly review where we are, what we are doing and what impact we are having, through the process of global public health diagnosis, treatment and follow-up.

AND FINALLY...

To confront the myriad challenges that comprise today's global public health crisis, we, the international public health community, need to do three things. First, we need to recognise that we face (now or in the near future) such a crisis; second, we need to plan and implement countermeasures in a systematic, evidence-based manner; third, we need to collect and analyse data that will enable us to monitor progress. It would be pointless to expend too much time and effort on that first step. I have argued in the course of this book that a global public health crisis is indeed upon us (or at least imminent) but this is a matter of judgement. We can predict neither the future with accuracy nor the time scale over which the emerging threats to global population health and wellbeing will unfold. Commentators will probably never agree on what constitutes a crisis and whether or not our current position merits that label. The argument is a semantic one. We may have to agree to disagree on both points and then move on.

It will be much more productive if we can all decide, as rapidly as possible, to use all the available data to make a global health diagnosis, to reach a consensus on what treatment to prescribe, and to draw up plans for the implementation and evaluation of interventions. What is not seriously in dispute is the overwhelming moral imperative to act collectively and resolutely to maximise the prospects of achieving the inspirational yet achievable vision of better health and wellbeing for all of humanity in the course of the 21st century.

A proposed 'horizontal' global public health strategy

Here are five principles, 20 goals and 60 related actions, with the top six priorities (*see* Chapter 10) highlighted in italics.

PRINCIPLE 1: EMBRACE A HOLISTIC APPROACH TO HEALTH AND DISEASE ON WHICH TO BASE PUBLIC HEALTH RESPONSES

Goal 1.1: ensure that physical, mental and social health dimensions are all integrated into public health strategies

Related actions
1 Include all three dimensions of health – physical, mental and social – into all public health policy and practice, whether in the fields of health protection, health improvement or healthcare management.
2 In assessing population health, include indicators of all three dimensions of health – physical, mental and social – in both the positive sense (well-being) and negative sense (absence of disease or disability).
3 *Adopt integrated, cross-cutting 'horizontal' approaches to public health policy and practice that seek to influence multiple health outcomes as well as adopting 'vertical' or single outcome approaches.*

Goal 1.2: seek salutogenic as well as anti-pathogenic solutions to public health challenges

Related actions
1 Nurture a salutogenic (health-promoting) as well as a pathogenic (disease causation) perspective on all aspects of public health policy and practice.
2 In addition to developing and implementing disease prevention measures, identify and promote resilience and related characteristics of individuals, families, communities and populations that promote and improve positive health.
3 *Pursue vigorous poverty reduction measures in recognition of the pathogenic role of poverty and the salutogenic role of affluence.*

Goal 1.3: promote the creation of safe, nurturing and sustainable environments as well as behavioural/lifestyle changes and good healthcare

Related actions

1   Recognise that the environment factors – physical, emotional and social – are at least as important as behaviour and healthcare in preventing disease and improving health.
2   *Shift the dominant focus of health improvement activity away from behavioural or lifestyle change and individualistic healthcare towards sustainable environmental modification.*
3   Expand the remit of health protection and environmental health beyond traditional concerns of pollution and infection to include the creation of safe, nurturing (salutogenic) and sustainable environments.

Goal 1.4: recognise and exploit the untapped potential of healthcare for the improvement of population health

Related actions

1   Discard divisive and unhelpful theoretical and practical distinctions between the work of public health and healthcare practitioners and policy makers.
2   Recognise the contribution of healthcare interventions (such as immunisation and screening) and systems to the achievement of public health objectives in the training and organisation of practitioners.
3   Integrate health improvement, health protection and healthcare practitioners and systems into public health policy making and practice.

PRINCIPLE 2: APPLY A PRAGMATIC EVIDENCE-BASED APPROACH TO PUBLIC HEALTH POLICY MAKING AND PRACTICE

Goal 2.1: use epidemiology to convert data into information, knowledge and understanding as well as to assess, monitor and address need

Related actions

1   Expand the use of epidemiological approaches to assess need, select appropriate interventions and evaluate progress.
2   *Build capacity in epidemiology to ensure that epidemiological and related data are appropriately analysed, interpreted and acted upon.*
3   Advocate greater use of 'shifting the distribution curve to the left' rather than 'targeting the tail' in the development of public health strategy development.

Goal 2.2: appraise evidence critically and systematically and disseminate the insights to practitioners and policy makers

Related actions

1 Secure strong commitment from the global public health community to an evidence-based approach to policy and practice.
2 Subject all existing and proposed public health policies, strategies, plans, programmes and other interventions to an 'evidence-based audit'.
3 Boost capacity in the critical appraisal of the research literature to facilitate the transfer of knowledge from researchers to practitioners.

Goal 2.3: take account of public perceptions without succumbing to popular prejudice

Related actions

1 Involve the general public, as key stakeholders, in the planning, delivery and evaluation or monitoring of all public health interventions.
2 Consult sensitively with vulnerable groups such as children, the elderly and other minorities, in the planning, delivery and evaluation or monitoring of all public health interventions.
3 Respond to reasonable public concerns about a public health intervention without jeopardising its beneficial impact.

Goal 2.4: generate new knowledge about health and disease by supporting goal-oriented public health research

Related actions

1 Identify major gaps in knowledge about the epidemiology, causes, treatment and prevention of diseases, as well as about health improvement, and commission appropriate goal-oriented research to fill them.
2 Develop mechanisms for knowledge transfer between public health researchers and practitioners via translational research and other forms of research dissemination.
3 Build public health research capacity through resource allocation, training and career development.

PRINCIPLE 3: ADOPT A LIFECOURSE APPROACH TO PUBLIC HEALTH ANALYSIS AND INTERVENTION

Goal 3.1: start early in the human life cycle, from preconception and intergenerationally where possible

Related actions

1 Adopt a long-term and intergenerational perspective on the assessment, intervention and monitoring of health across the lifecourse.

2 Focus specific attention on the practical and emotional needs of parents (especially mothers), children and families in the early part of the lifecourse.
3 Seek to minimise the occurrence, severity and impact of adverse childhood experiences – physical, emotional and social – in early life.

Goal 3.2: sustain effort throughout the lifecourse unremittingly to the end of life

Related actions

1 Integrate public health policies and practices aimed at specific objectives or age groups (such as health inequality reduction and chronic risk factor disease control) across the lifecourse.
2 Ensure that early interventions (in pregnancy, infancy and childhood) are reinforced by later ones to avoid attenuating long-term gains.
3 Focus attention on especially vulnerable stages of the lifecourse – especially the very early and very late stages – when the potential for effective intervention is greatest.

Goal 3.3: reprioritise attention and resources from later to earlier in the lifecourse

Related actions

1 Advocate early intervention as an evidence-based public health strategy for the improvement of health and prevention of disease.
2 Undertake cost–benefit and other economic analyses of the likely financial return on investment in the early part of the lifecourse.
3 *Shift health-promoting resources and capacity from later to earlier parts of the lifecourse without causing serious detriment to older age groups.*

Goal 3.4: incorporate lifecourse approaches to all forms of health inequality (social, gender, ethnic, geographical) reduction

Related actions

1 Identify commonalities and divergences between different forms of health inequality across the lifecourse.
2 Implement health inequality reduction strategies and interventions across the entire lifecourse.
3 Seek to minimise the impact of poverty, and other causes of health inequality, on the most vulnerable age groups, especially children and the elderly.

PRINCIPLE 4: CREATE EFFICIENT AND TRANSPARENT GOVERNANCE PROCESSES FOR PUBLIC HEALTH ACTION

Goal 4.1: create robust ethical and legal frameworks for public health policy making and practice

Related actions

1   Subject public health practitioners to an ethical code of practice as robust as that applicable to doctors and other healthcare professionals.
2   Strive for an international consensus on the nature of the ethical and legal rights and obligations of public health practitioners.
3   Seek legal protection for public health practitioners who may encounter pressures, threats and other barriers to their pursuit of legitimate public health objectives.

Goal 4.2: take account of financial costs and benefits of potential interventions

Related actions

1   Include health econometric approaches – especially cost–benefit analyses – into strategic public health planning.
2   Increase health economic capacity in academic and service departments of public health.
3   Resist the use of exclusively or predominantly economic arguments or data on which to base public health decision making.

Goal 4.3: create appropriate mechanisms for delivering and monitoring intersectoral public health.

Related actions

1   Seek high-level policy endorsement for intersectoral, multidisciplinary working as the norm for all public health activity.
2   Incorporate intersectoral, multidisciplinary working into job descriptions and appraisal processes across the public health workforce.
3   Develop administrative delivery structures, backed by adequate resources, to plan, implement and monitor public health interventions including those requiring rapid responses to acute (including infectious, environmental or humanitarian) incidents.

Goal 4.4: boost high-quality public health capacity through standardised, affordable and practical education, training and career development

Related actions

1   Highlight the need for an expanded multidisciplinary workforce throughout the world to deliver improvements in global health.

2   Inspire, recruit and retain to the public health workforce through high-quality undergraduate and postgraduate training.
3   Provide appropriate, standardised, affordable and practical educational courses, training programmes, and career structures for the public health workforce.

PRINCIPLE 5: STRIVE FOR A COMPREHENSIVE STRATEGIC APPROACH TO PUBLIC HEALTH POLICY MAKING AND PRACTICE

Goal 5.1: identify, nurture and promote leadership and advocacy for public health across all professions and sectors

Related actions
1   Provide additional training to suitably motivated and talented individuals to enable them to adopt leadership roles within multidisciplinary and multisectoral public health.
2   Allocate clearly defined leadership roles to sectors, agencies and individuals to facilitate public health policy making and practice.
3   Enhance public health advocacy in all relevant spheres of both public and private sector policy and practice.

Goal 5.2: forge strategic alliances with non-health sectors responsible for health-relevant policies such as those concerned with the economy, climate change and security

Related actions
1   Establish effective mechanisms for collaboration between health and non-health sectors in pursuit of public health objectives.
2   Secure a cross-sectoral consensus that the improvement and protection of population health represent an important strategic policy objective.
3   Ensure that health is widely viewed across government departments and beyond as both an end in itself and as a necessary input to economic development, countering climate change, national security and other strategic objectives.

Goal 5.3: work globally to achieve public health objectives internationally, regionally, nationally and locally

Related actions
1   Raise awareness of the transnational nature of contemporary threats to population health and the need to mount global as well as national and local responses.

2 Building on existing organisations, strengthen the global public health infrastructure to optimise international co-operation and collaboration to address global health challenges.
3 *Seek to integrate the various international statements, agreements, strategies and programmes into a single, overarching, streamlined global public health strategy.*

Goal 5.4: incorporate evaluation and the capacity to change into all public health activity

Related actions
1 Stress the ethical and practical imperative to evaluate all public health interventions to ensure that precious public resources are invested in the most effective and efficient manner possible.
2 Enhance evaluational capacity through undergraduate, postgraduate and in-service training of students and practitioners.
3 Ensure that the necessary feedback loops are constructed to enable public health staff to respond appropriately to the results of evaluation and monitoring.

Index